MUSCLES & NERVES

An Ultrasound Tracing Atlas

Labeled Sonograms for Anatomical Identification

Forearm Wrist Hand

AF896470

HAJIME TSUCHIDA

Sonographer, Australia

Collaborator: Palmu Sherpa
Sonographer, Australia

Copyright© 2025 by Hajime Tsuchida. All rights reserved.

No part of this publication may be reproduced, distributed, or transmitted in any form or by any means, including photocopying, recording, or other electronic or mechanical methods, without written permission from the author, except as permitted under the copyright law.

Cover design: James T. Egan of Bookfly Design

Interior design: Scott Moden

Disclaimer

The information contained in this book may not be accurate or complete. Neither the author nor the publisher guarantees its accuracy or completeness and shall not be held liable for any damages arising from actions taken based on its contents.

This book is intended for educational and reference purposes only. The author is a qualified sonographer. The content should not be used as a substitute for professional medical diagnosis or treatment. Always consult a professional before acting on any information within this publication.

Contents

Preface

The field of ultrasonographic anatomy for muscles and peripheral nerves is still evolving, and a systematic approach for the depiction and interpretation of these structures has yet to be fully established. Nevertheless, increasing international interest in this area has contributed to a steady accumulation of new knowledge and clinical insight.

The ability to visualize muscles and peripheral nerves through ultrasound offers significant benefits across many medical specialties. Furthermore, the capacity to observe internal structures dynamically and non-invasively is a feature of ultrasound that continues to hold strong scientific and clinical appeal.

This volume presents a record of the author's exploratory work within a largely uncharted domain. It is intended to support readers in deepening their understanding and advancing their work in this field. While some uncertainties may remain within these pages, the content is offered with the expectation that it will provide practical and meaningful information for clinicians, sonographers, and educators with an interest in the ultrasonographic anatomy of muscles and peripheral nerves.

I would also like to express my profound gratitude to the many experts around the world whose guidance and contributions have played a vital role in bringing this book to completion. It is my sincere hope that this work will help readers gain clearer insight into this field and contribute, even in a small way, to future research, education, and clinical development.

SECTION 1

Fig. 1 Radial Fossa / Coronoid Fossa

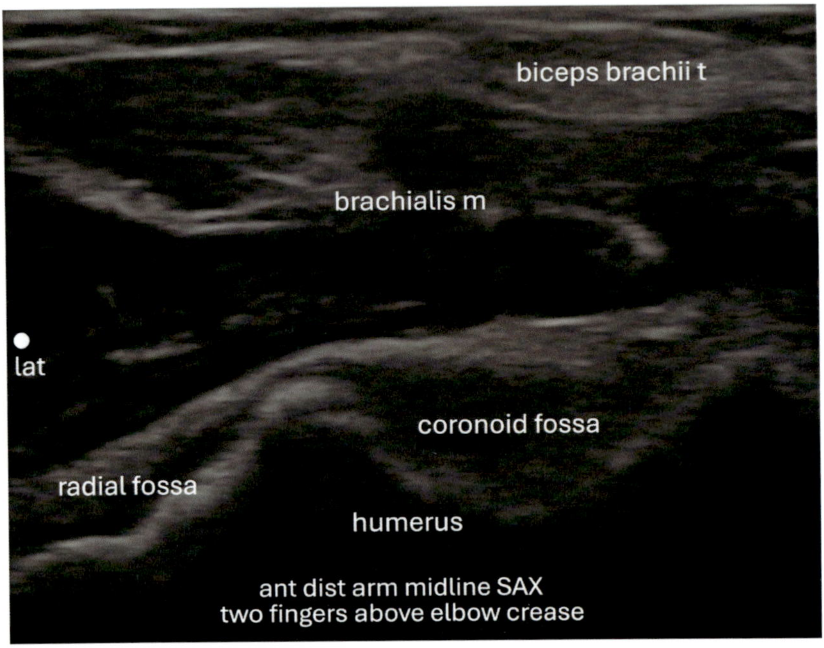

Probe Position: The probe is placed transversely (with its axis perpendicular to the arm) along the midline of the anterior distal arm, approximately two fingerbreadths above the elbow crease.

Anatomical Landmark: The coronoid fossa of the humerus.

Visualized Structures: Both the coronoid fossa and the radial fossa of the humerus are visualized.

Other Structures: The biceps brachii tendon and the brachialis muscle are also visible.

Fig. 2 Articular Cartilage of Anterior Elbow Capitulum / Trochlea of Humerus

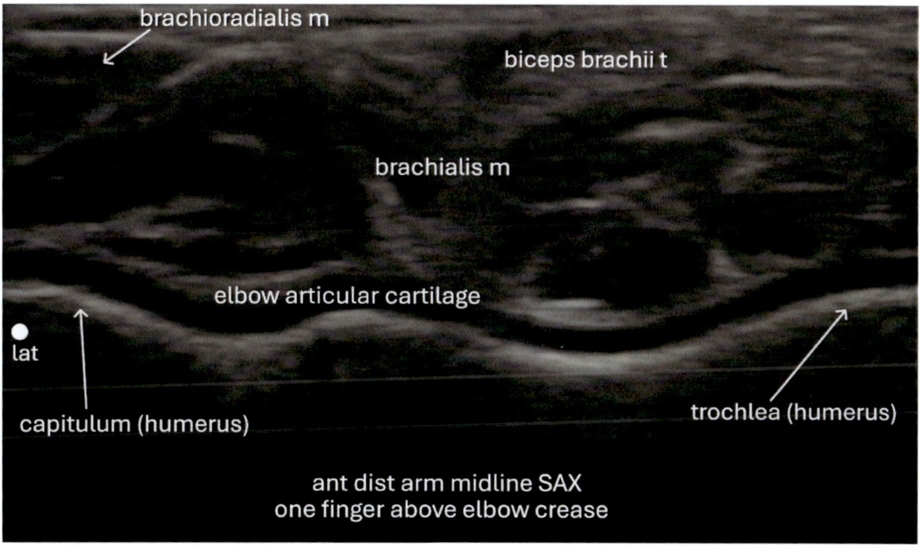

Probe Position: The probe is placed transversely along the midline of the anterior distal arm, approximately one fingerbreadth above the elbow crease, just distal to the position shown in Fig. 1.

Anatomical Landmark: The articular cartilage of the anterior elbow.

Visualized Structures: The trochlea and capitulum of the humerus are visualized beneath the articular cartilage of the anterior elbow.

Other Structures: The biceps brachii tendon, as well as the brachialis and brachioradialis muscles, are also visible.

Fig. 3 Radial Head / Coronoid Process of Ulna

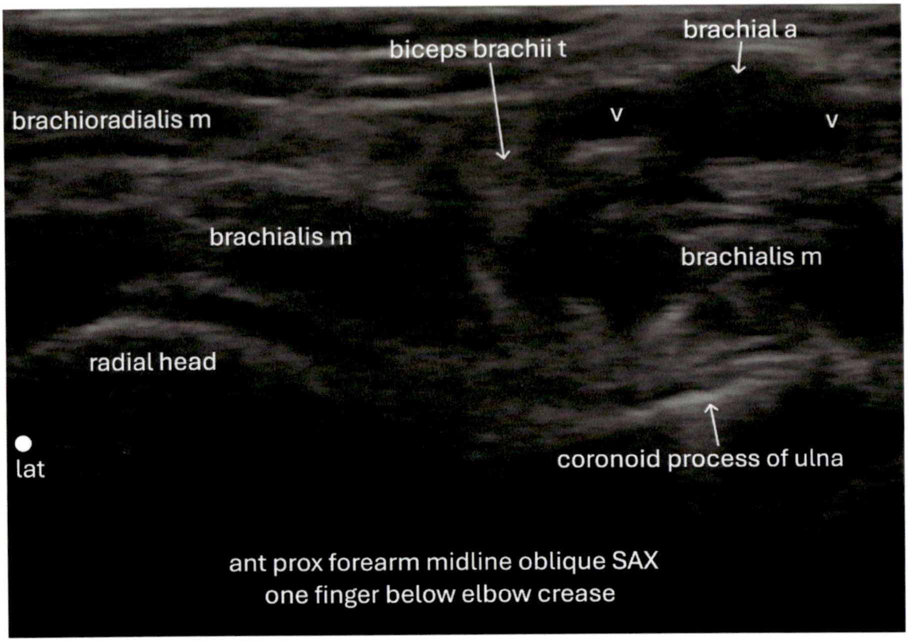

Probe Position: The probe is placed transversely, but slightly obliquely, along the midline of the anterior proximal forearm, approximately one fingerbreadth below the elbow crease, just distal to the position shown in Fig. 2.

Anatomical Landmarks: The ulna and the radius.

Visualized Structures: The coronoid process of the ulna and the radial head can be visualized side by side in a single view by slightly rotating the probe so that the ulnar side of the probe is positioned slightly superior to the radial side.

Other Structures: The biceps brachii tendon, the brachialis, and the brachioradialis muscles are visible. The brachial artery and veins can also be seen.

Fig. 4 Longitudinal View
Radial Fossa / Capitulum / Radial Head

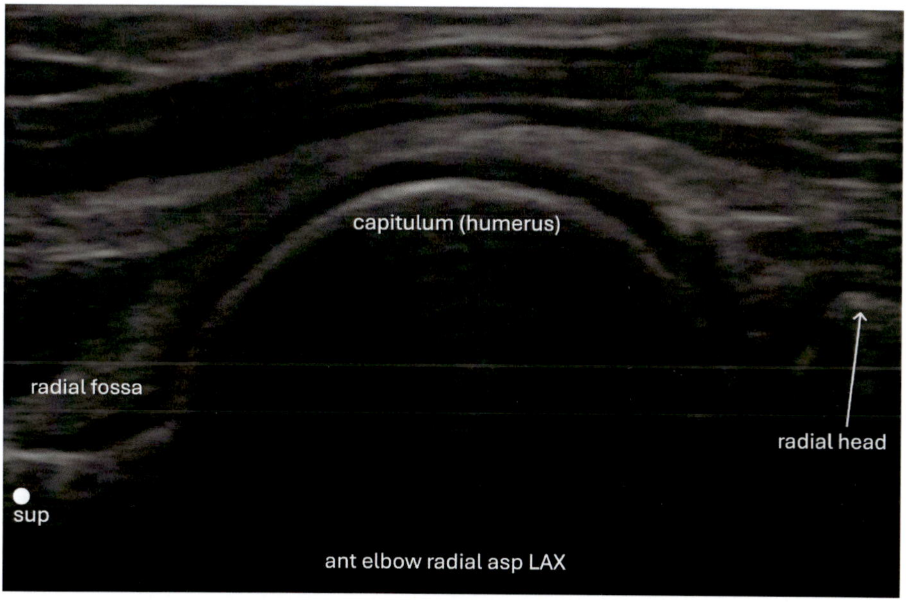

Probe Position: The probe is placed longitudinally on the radial aspect of the anterior elbow.

Anatomical Landmarks: The humerus and the radius.

Visualized Structures: The radial fossa, capitulum, and radial head are visualized in the longitudinal view.

Other Structure: The articular cartilage of the anterior elbow is also visible.

Fig. 5 Longitudinal View Coronoid Fossa / Trochlea / Coronoid Process of Ulna

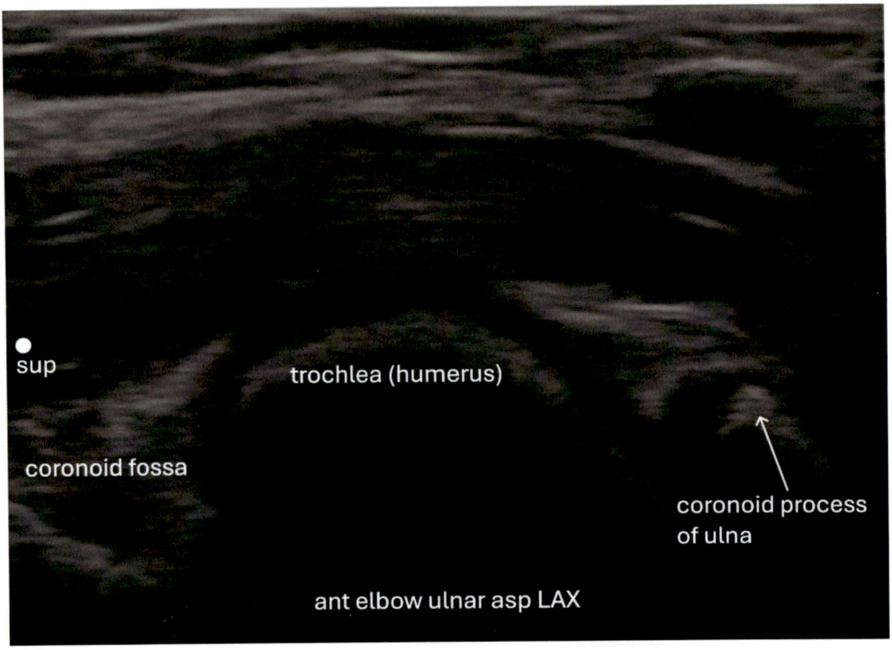

Probe Position: The probe is placed longitudinally on the ulnar aspect of the anterior elbow.

Anatomical Landmarks: The humerus and the ulna.

Visualized Structures: The coronoid fossa, trochlea, and coronoid process of the ulna are visualized in the longitudinal view.

Other Structure: The articular cartilage of the anterior elbow is also visible.

SECTION 2

Fig. 1 Articular Cartilage of Anterior Elbow / Median Nerve

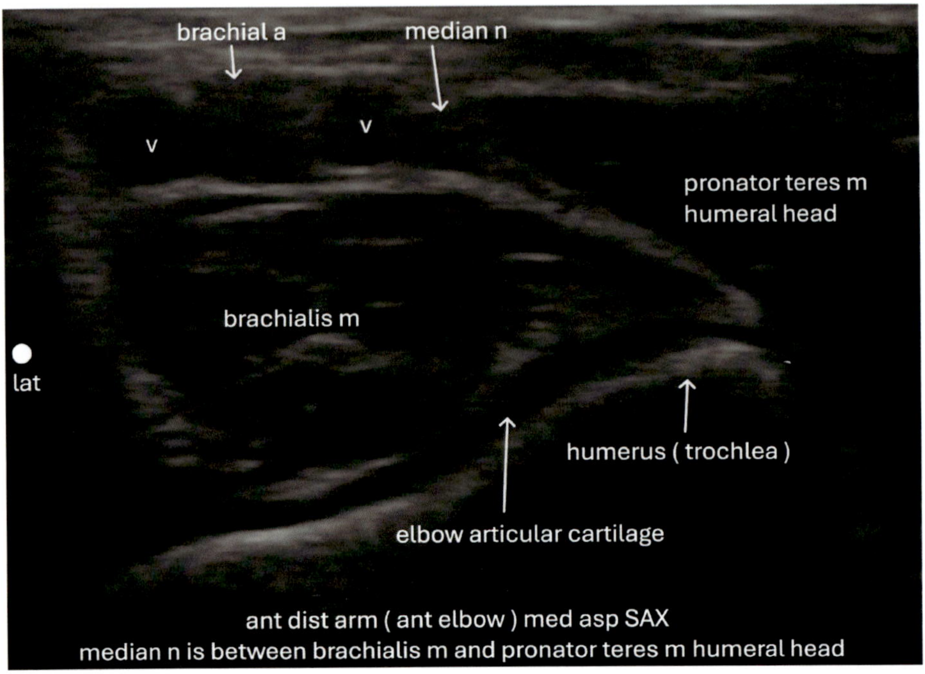

Probe Position: The probe is placed transversely (with its axis perpendicular to the arm) immediately proximal to the ulnar side of the elbow crease.

Anatomical Landmark: The anterior elbow articular cartilage at the trochlea of the humerus.

Surrounding Structures: The median nerve is surrounded by the brachial vein, the humeral head of the pronator teres muscle, and the brachialis muscle.

Other Structures: The anterior elbow articular cartilage and the trochlea of the humerus are also visible.

Fig. 2 Median Nerve / Coronoid Process of Ulna

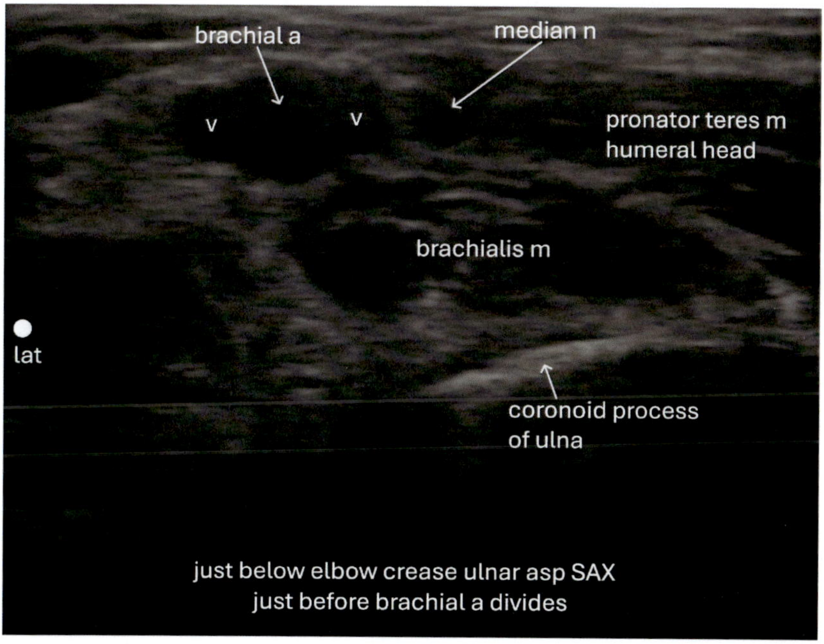

Probe Position: The probe is placed transversely just distal to the elbow crease on the ulnar side, immediately distal to the position shown in Fig. 1.

Anatomical Landmark: The coronoid process of the ulna.

Surrounding Structures: The median nerve is surrounded by the brachial vein, the humeral head of the pronator teres muscle, and the brachialis muscle.

Other Structure: The coronoid process of the ulna is visualized deep to the brachialis muscle.

Fig. 3 Median Nerve / Ulnar Artery / Ulnar Vein

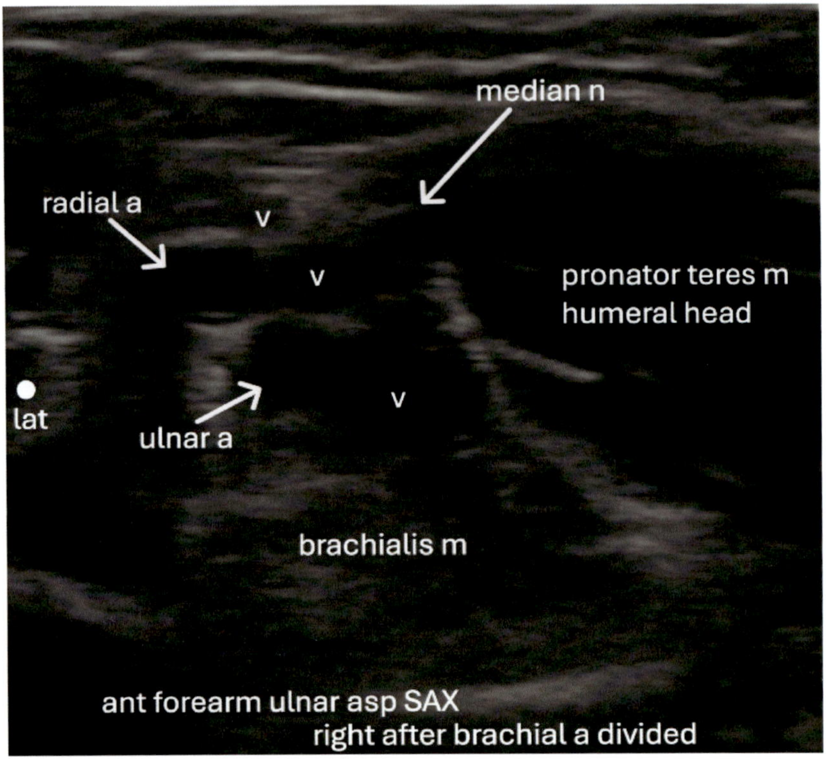

Probe Position: The probe is placed transversely on the ulnar side of the proximal forearm, immediately distal to the position shown in Fig. 2.

Anatomical Landmarks: The ulnar artery and vein.

Surrounding Structures: The median nerve is surrounded by the ulnar artery and vein, and the humeral head of the pronator teres muscle.

Additional Observation: The brachial artery divides into the radial artery and the ulnar artery.

Fig. 4 Median Nerve / Ulnar Artery / Ulnar Vein

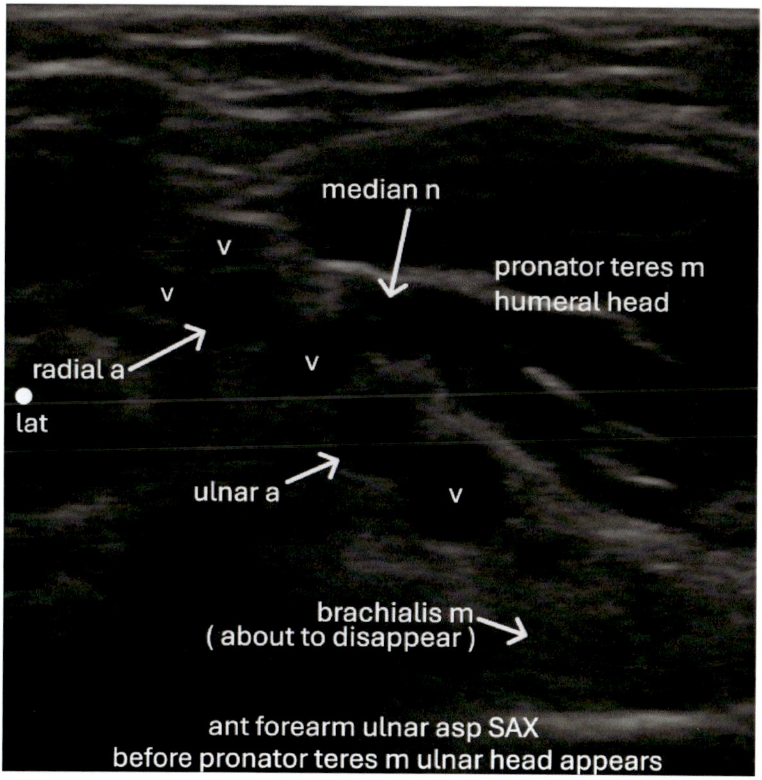

Probe Position: The probe is placed transversely on the ulnar side of the proximal forearm, immediately distal to the position shown in Fig. 3.

Anatomical Landmarks: The ulnar artery and vein.

Surrounding Structures: The median nerve is surrounded by the ulnar artery and vein, and the humeral head of the pronator teres muscle.

Additional Observation: As the transducer is moved slightly distally from this position, the brachialis muscle can no longer be visualized.

Fig. 5 Median Nerve / Ulnar Head of Pronator Teres Muscle

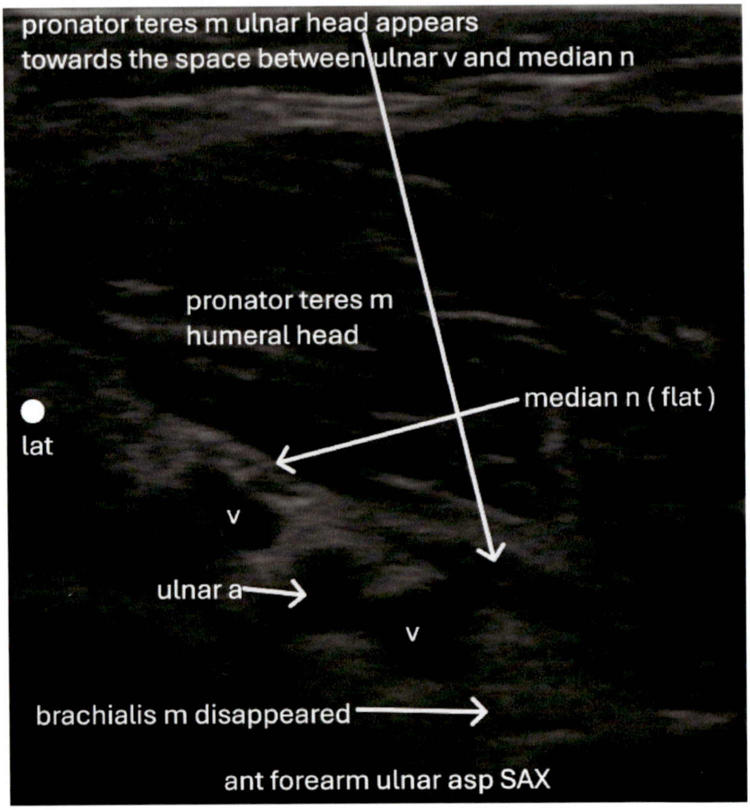

Probe Position: The probe is placed transversely on the ulnar side of the proximal forearm, immediately distal to the position shown in Fig. 4.

Anatomical Landmark: The ulnar head of the pronator teres muscle.

Surrounding Structures: The median nerve is located between the ulnar vein and the humeral head of the pronator teres muscle.

Additional Observation: The brachialis muscle moves out of view towards its insertion as the ulnar head of the pronator teres muscle comes into view.

Fig. 6 Median Nerve / Ulnar Head of Pronator Teres Muscle

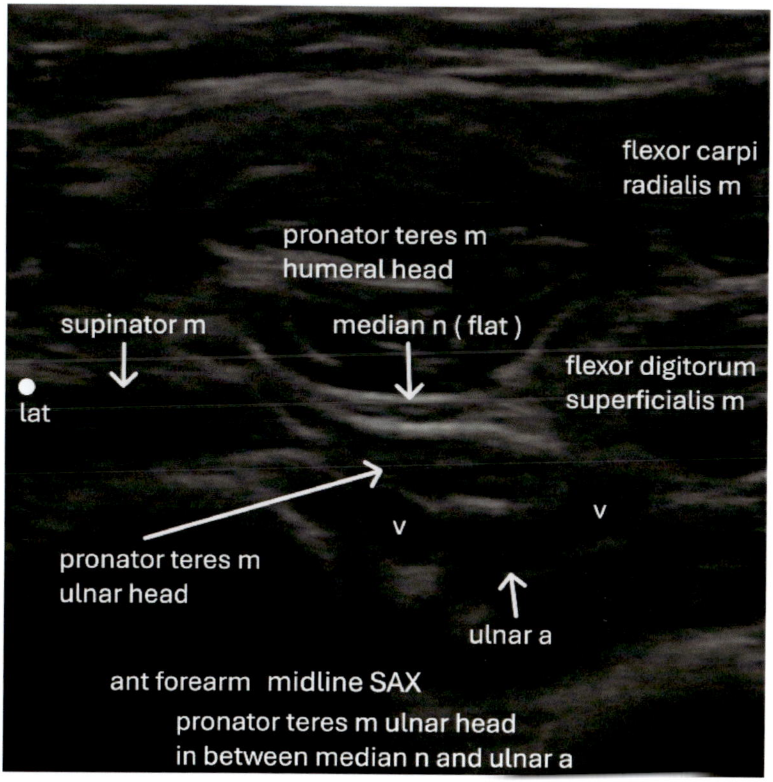

Probe Position: The probe is placed transversely on the midline of the proximal forearm, immediately distal to the location shown in Fig. 5.

Anatomical Landmark: The ulnar head of the pronator teres muscle.

Surrounding Structures: The median nerve is situated between the ulnar head and the humeral head of the pronator teres muscle.

Additional Observations: The ulnar head of the pronator teres muscle is visualized between the median nerve and the ulnar vein. The median nerve appears flattened in this short segment. Additionally, the supinator muscle begins to become visible on the radial side.

Fig. 7 Median Nerve / Ulnar Head of Pronator Teres Muscle

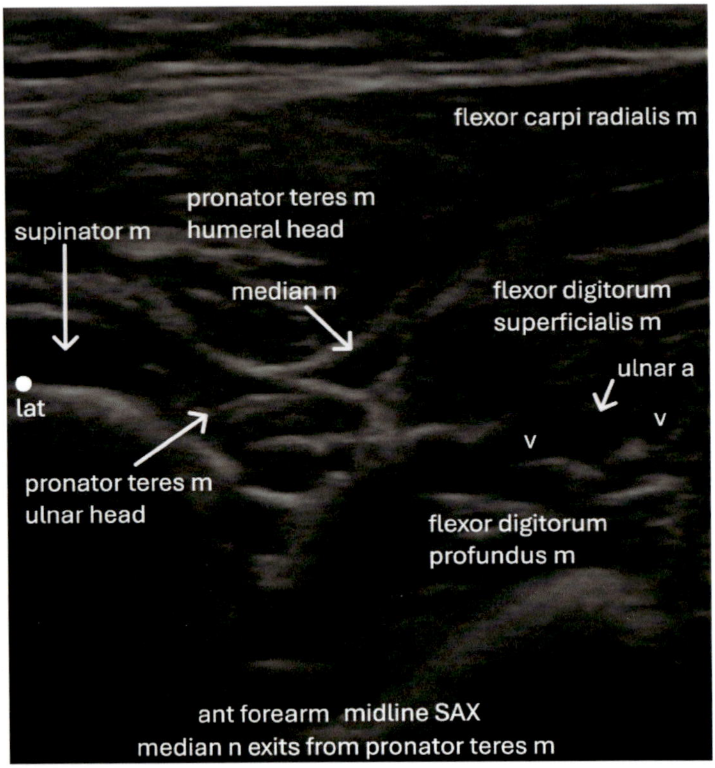

Probe Position: The probe is placed transversely on the midline of the proximal forearm, immediately distal to the location shown in Fig. 6.

Anatomical Landmark: The ulnar head of the pronator teres muscle.

Surrounding Structures: The median nerve is surrounded by the ulnar head and the humeral head of the pronator teres muscle, as well as the humeroulnar head of the flexor digitorum superficialis muscle.

Additional Observations: The median nerve exits between the two heads of the pronator teres muscle. The image also shows the ulnar artery distal to the origin of the common interosseous artery, which then branches into the anterior and posterior interosseous arteries. Additionally, the flexor digitorum profundus muscle becomes evident. The anterior interosseous nerve also originates from the deep side of the median nerve around this level.

Fig. 8 Median Nerve / Sublime Bridge / Radial Head of Flexor Digitorum Superficialis Muscle

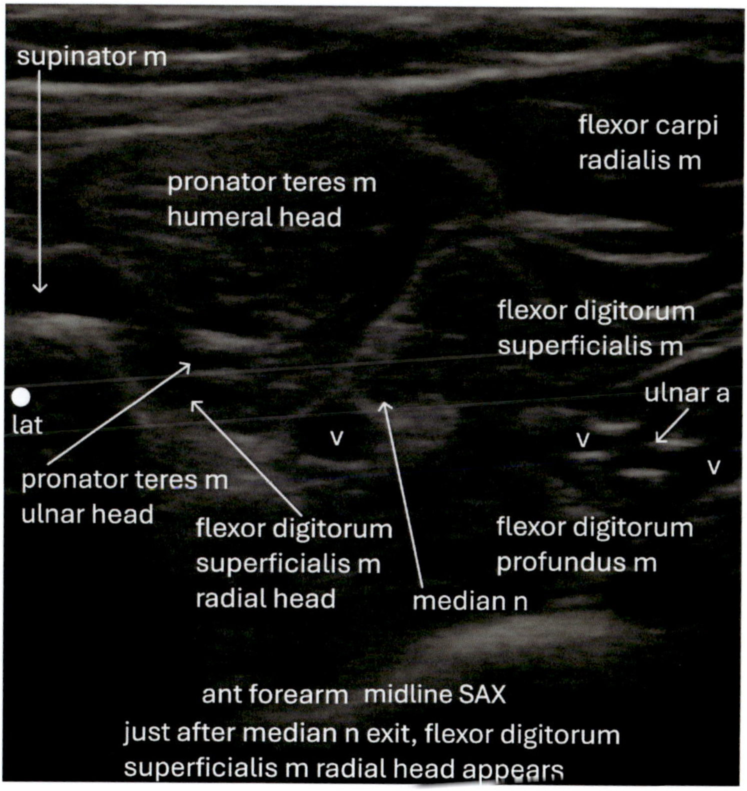

Probe Position: The probe is placed transversely on the midline of the proximal forearm, immediately distal to the location shown in Fig. 7.

Anatomical Landmark: The fibrous arch of the flexor digitorum superficialis muscle (The sublime bridge).

Surrounding Structures: The median nerve is deep to the sublime bridge, which is located between the radial head of the flexor digitorum superficialis muscle and the humeroulnar head of the flexor digitorum superficialis muscle.

Additional Observation: On the radial bone, the radial head of the flexor digitorum superficialis muscle begins to appear deep to the ulnar head of the pronator teres muscle, which will soon move out of view.

Fig. 9 Median Nerve / Anterior Interosseous Nerve / Flexor Pollicis Longus Muscle

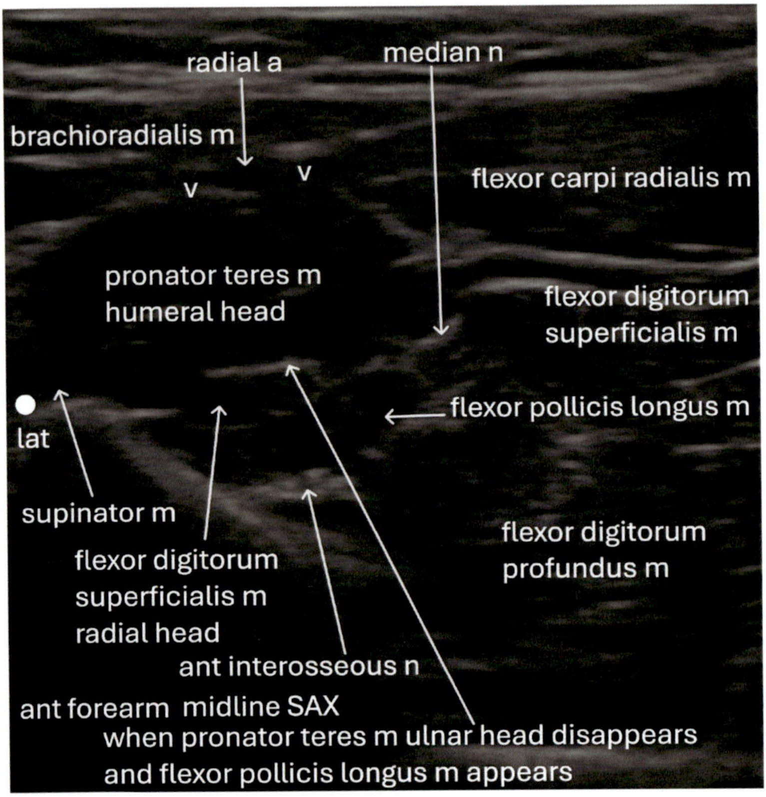

Probe Position: The probe is placed transversely over the midline of the mid-forearm, just below the area indicated in Fig. 8.

Anatomical Landmark: The flexor pollicis longus muscle.

Surrounding Structures: The median nerve is located between the flexor pollicis longus muscle and the humeroulnar head of the flexor digitorum superficialis muscle.

Additional Observations: The flexor pollicis longus muscle starts to emerge deep to the radial head of the flexor digitorum superficialis muscle on the radial bone. The ulnar head of the pronator teres muscle is no longer in view. The anterior interosseous nerve can be seen between the flexor pollicis longus muscle and the flexor digitorum profundus muscle.

Fig. 10 Median Nerve / Anterior Interosseous Nerve / Flexor Pollicis Longus Muscle

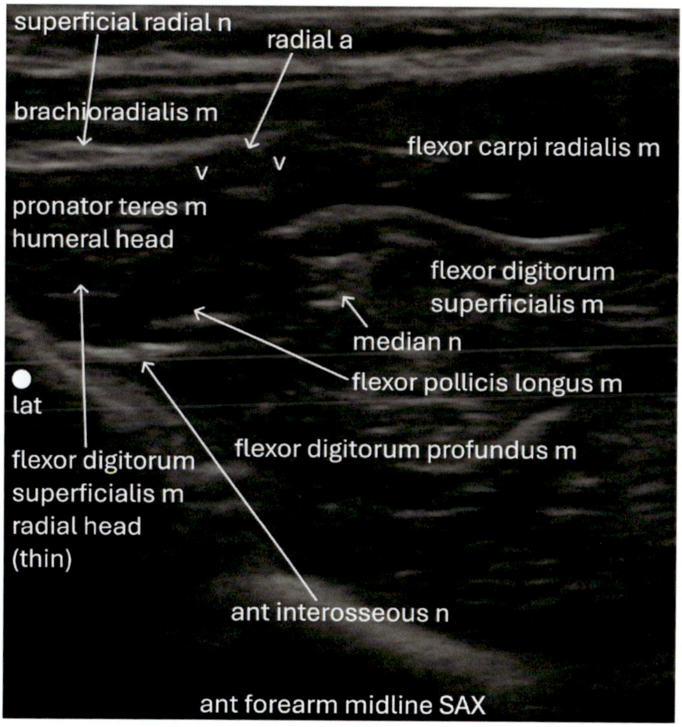

Probe Position: The probe is placed transversely over the midline of the mid-forearm, just below the area indicated in Fig. 9.

Anatomical Landmark: The flexor pollicis longus muscle.

Surrounding Structures: The median nerve is located between the flexor pollicis longus muscle and the humeroulnar head of the flexor digitorum superficialis muscle.

Additional Observations: The anterior interosseous nerve can be seen between the flexor pollicis longus muscle and the flexor digitorum profundus muscle. Identifying these individual muscles in the image can be aided by performing their specific actions:

- Flexor pollicis longus: flexes the interphalangeal joint of the thumb.
- Flexor digitorum profundus: flexes the distal interphalangeal joints.
- Flexor digitorum superficialis: flexes the proximal interphalangeal joints.

Fig. 11 Median Nerve / Anterior Interosseous Nerve / Flexor Pollicis Longus Muscle

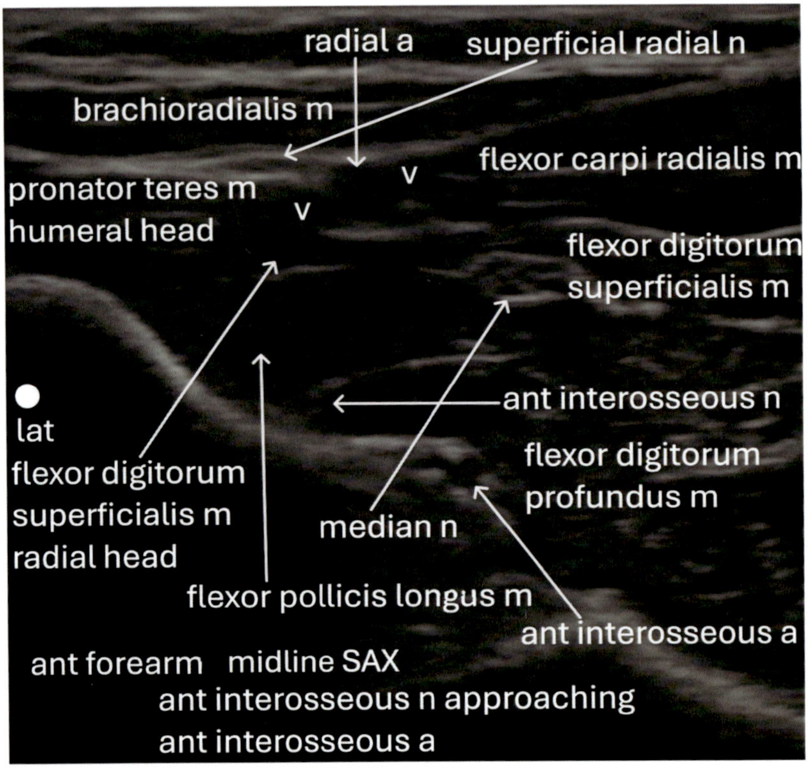

Probe Position: The probe is placed transversely over the midline of the mid-forearm, just below the area indicated in Fig. 10.

Anatomical Landmark: The flexor pollicis longus muscle.

Surrounding Structures: The median nerve is located between the flexor pollicis longus muscle and the humeroulnar head of the flexor digitorum superficialis muscle.

Additional Observations: The anterior interosseous nerve is situated between the flexor pollicis longus and flexor digitorum profundus muscles. Furthermore, the anterior interosseous nerve is seen approaching the anterior interosseous vein. In this view, there is a reduction in the size of the humeral head of the pronator teres muscle.

Fig. 12 Median Nerve / Anterior Interosseous Nerve / Flexor Pollicis Longus Muscle

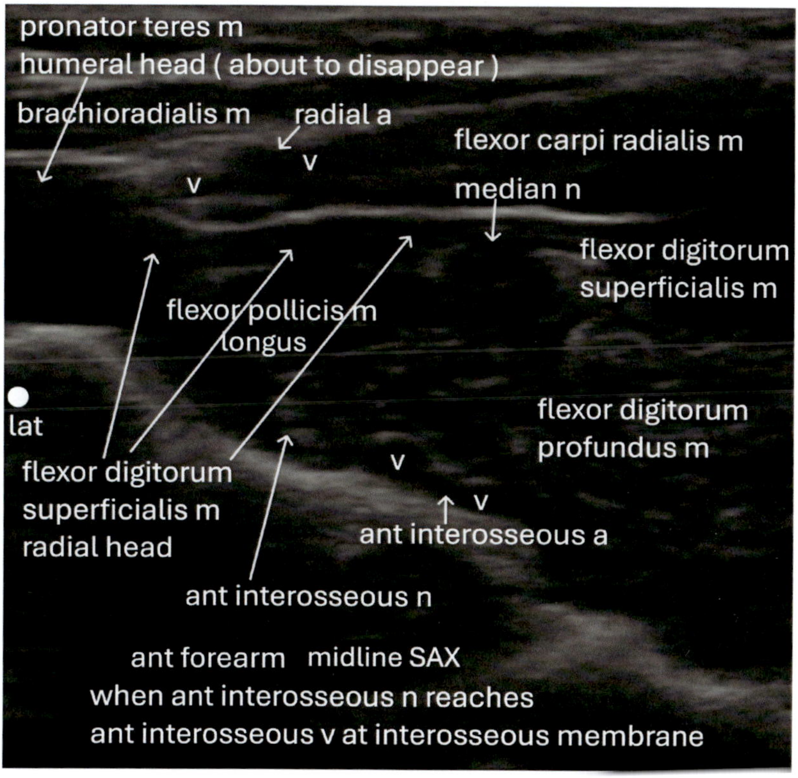

Probe Position: The probe is placed transversely over the midline of the mid-forearm, just below the area indicated in Fig. 11.

Anatomical Landmarks: The anterior interosseous artery and vein.

Surrounding Structures: The median nerve is located between the flexor pollicis longus muscle and the humeroulnar head of the flexor digitorum superficialis muscle.

Additional Observations: The anterior interosseous nerve is situated between the flexor pollicis longus and flexor digitorum profundus muscles. Furthermore, the anterior interosseous nerve is seen to be in close proximity to the anterior interosseous vein on the anterior aspect of the interosseous membrane, which lies between the radius and ulna bones in the forearm. At this level, the humeral head of the pronator teres muscle is soon going out of view.

Fig. 13 Median Nerve / Flexor Pollicis Longus Muscle

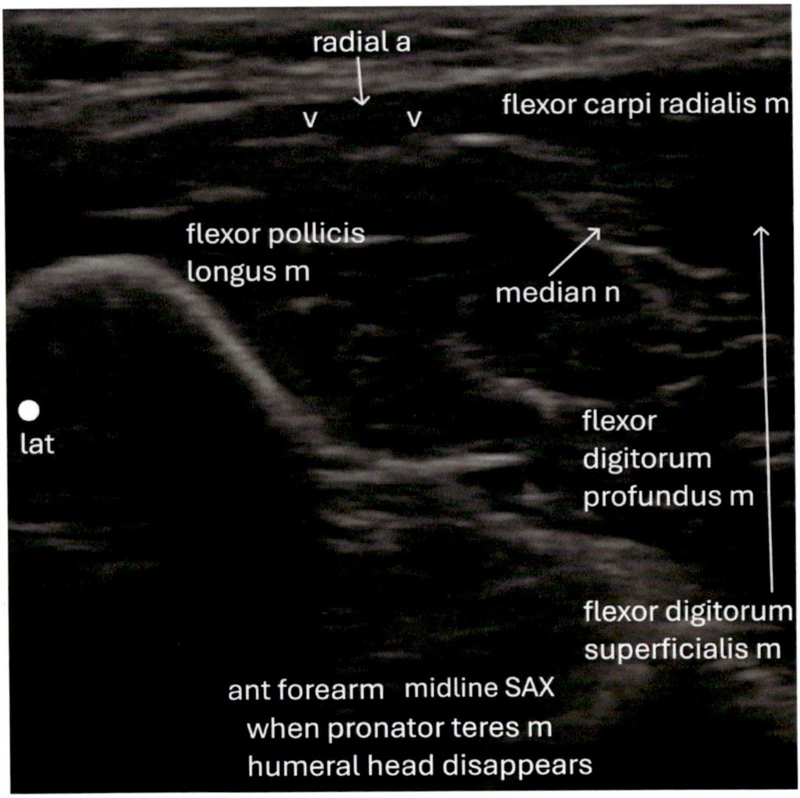

Probe Position: The probe is placed transversely over the midline of the mid-forearm, just distal to the area indicated in Fig. 12.

Anatomical Landmark: The flexor pollicis longus muscle.

Surrounding Structures: The median nerve is located between the flexor pollicis longus muscle and the humeroulnar head of the flexor digitorum superficialis muscle.

Additional Observation: The humeral head of the pronator teres muscle moved out of view for its insertion to the radius.

Fig. 14 Median Nerve / Musculotendinous Junction of Flexor Carpi Radialis

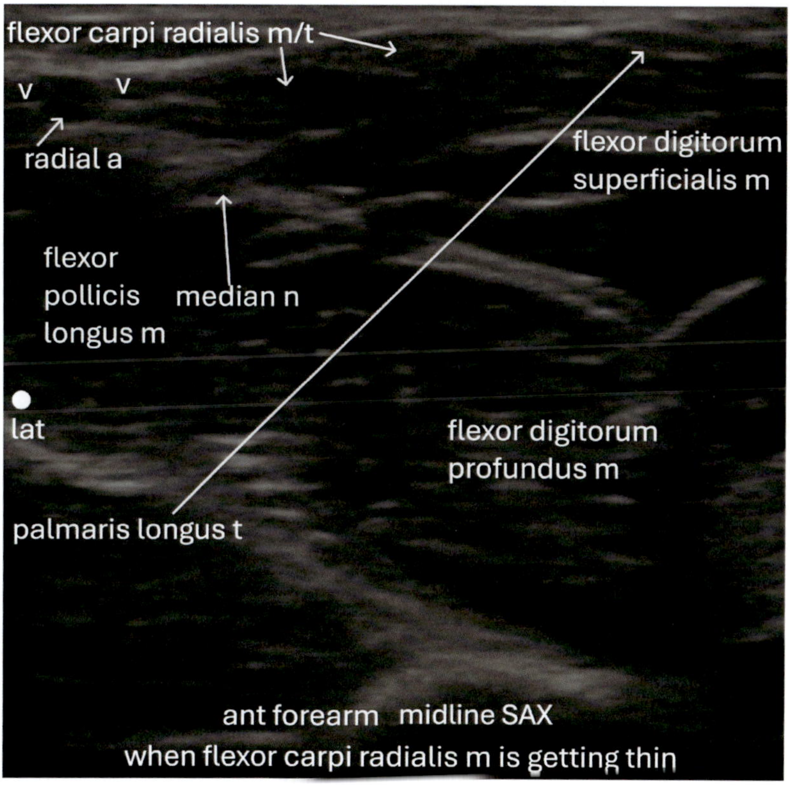

Probe Position: The probe is placed transversely over the midline of the distal forearm, just distal to the area indicated in Fig. 13.

Anatomical Landmark: The flexor pollicis longus muscle.

Surrounding Structures: The median nerve is located between the flexor pollicis longus muscle and the humeroulnar head of the flexor digitorum superficialis muscle.

Additional Observations: The palmaris longus tendon and the musculotendinous junction of the flexor carpi radialis muscle are superficially visible.

Fig. 15 Median Nerve / Flexor Carpi Radialis Tendon / Musculotendinous Junction of Flexor Pollicis Longus

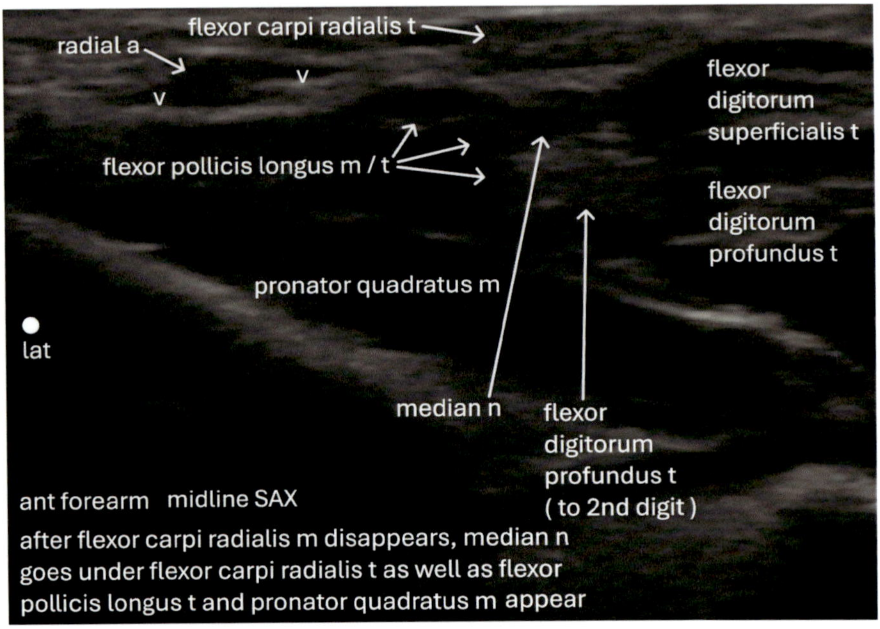

Probe Position: The probe is placed transversely over the midline of the distal forearm, just distal to the area indicated in Fig. 14.

Anatomical Landmarks: The flexor carpi radialis tendon and the distal part of the pronator quadratus muscle.

Surrounding Structures: Just deep to the flexor carpi radialis tendon, the median nerve can be seen. Just beneath the median nerve, two structures become visible: the flexor pollicis longus tendon laterally and the flexor digitorum profundus tendon for the second digit medially.

Additional Observations: The musculotendinous junctions of the flexor digitorum superficialis muscle and the flexor digitorum profundus muscle are visible at this level.

Fig. 16 Palmar Cutaneous Branch of Median Nerve / Median Nerve / Flexor Carpi Radialis Tendon / Flexor Pollicis Longus Tendon

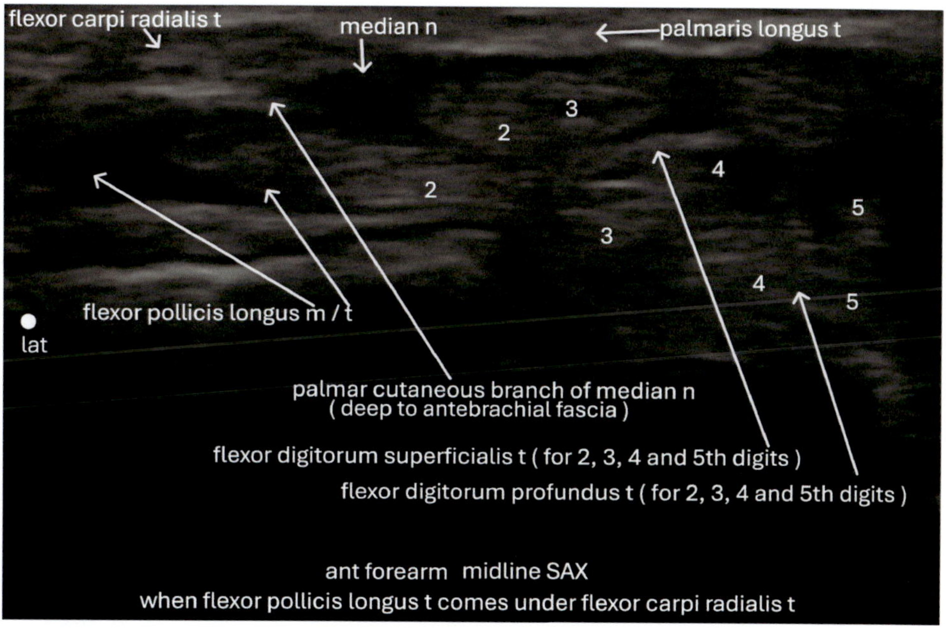

Probe Position: The probe is placed transversely over the midline of the distal forearm, just distal to the area indicated in Fig. 15.

Anatomical Landmarks: The flexor carpi radialis tendon and the flexor pollicis longus tendon

Surrounding Structures: The median nerve lies just deep to and at the medial edge of the flexor carpi radialis tendon. The palmar cutaneous branch of the median nerve, which is situated just deep to the antebrachial fascia at this level, can be seen just lateral to the median nerve, between the flexor carpi radialis tendon and the flexor pollicis longus tendon.

Additional Observations: This image shows the level where the pronator quadratus muscle is going out of view. The flexor digitorum superficialis tendons and the flexor digitorum profundus tendons for the 2nd to 5th digits are individually visible at this level. Identifying these individual tendons in the image can be aided by performing their specific actions.

Fig. 17 Palmar Cutaneous Branch of Median Nerve / Median Nerve / Flexor Carpi Radialis Tendon / Flexor Pollicis Longus Tendon

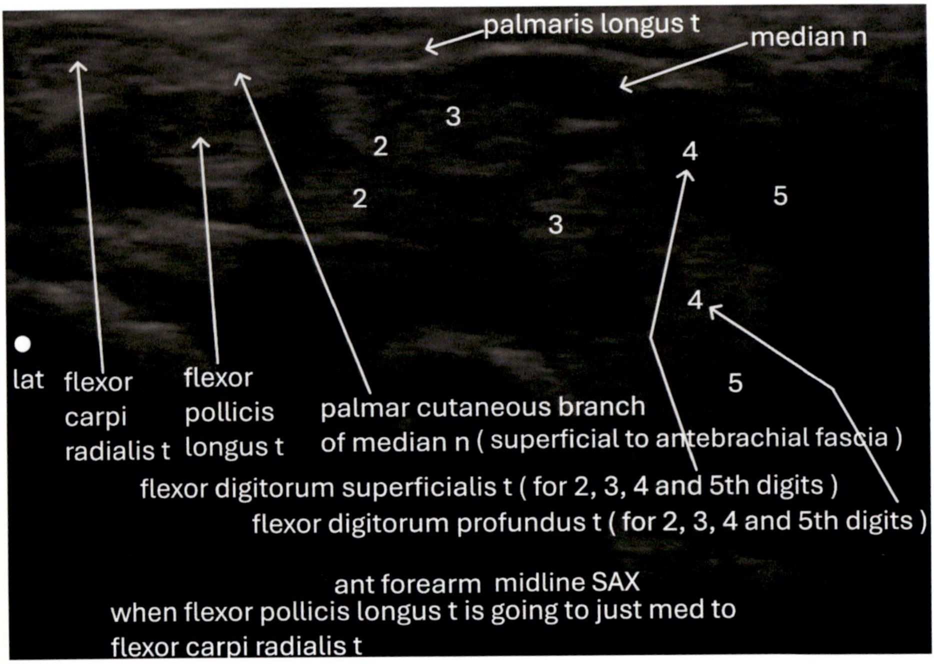

Probe Position: The probe is placed transversely over the midline of the distal forearm, just distal to the area indicated in Fig. 16.

Anatomical Landmarks: The flexor carpi radialis tendon and the flexor pollicis longus tendon.

Surrounding Structures: When the medial edge of the flexor pollicis longus tendon is slightly more medial to the medial edge of the flexor carpi radialis tendon, the palmar cutaneous branch of the median nerve, which is situated just superficial to the antebrachial fascia at this level, can be seen superficial to the medial part of the flexor pollicis longus tendon and just medial to the flexor carpi radialis tendon, while the median nerve passes medially into the superficial space, either between the second and third or between the third and fourth tendons of the flexor digitorum superficialis.

Additional Observations: At this level, the palmar cutaneous branch of the median nerve can be seen penetrating the antebrachial fascia from deep to superficial. Immediately distal to this point, it comes to lie on the superficial aspect of the thicker flexor retinaculum.

Fig. 18 Median Nerve / Proximal Carpal Tunnel / Scaphoid / Pisiform / Flexor Retinaculum

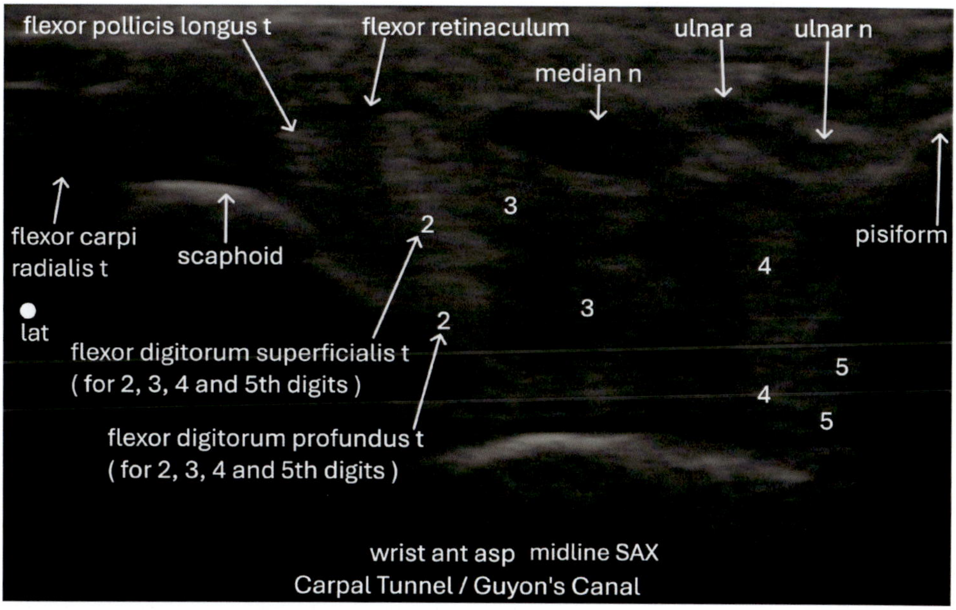

Probe Position: The probe is placed transversely over the midline of the anterior wrist, just distal to the area indicated in Fig. 17.

Anatomical Landmarks: The scaphoid and pisiform bones.

Surrounding Structures: The median nerve is located in the superficial space, between the third and fourth tendons of the flexor digitorum superficialis. The ulnar nerve can be seen in Guyon's Canal, between the ulnar artery and the pisiform bone.

Additional Observations: This image displays the proximal carpal tunnel, Guyon's Canal, and the flexor retinaculum.

Fig. 19 Median Nerve / Proximal Carpal Tunnel / Scaphoid / Flexor Carpi Radialis Tendon / Flexor Retinaculum

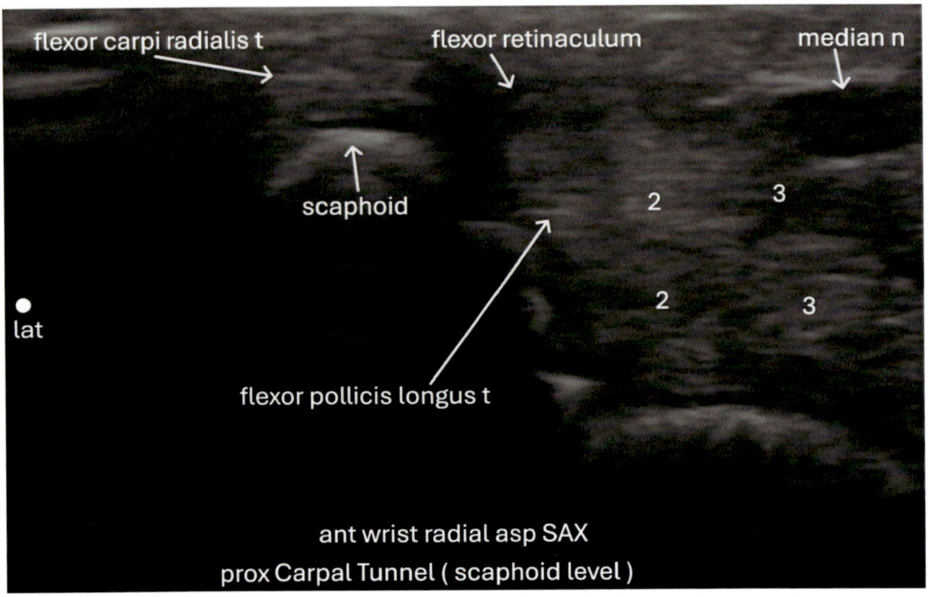

Probe Position: The probe is placed transversely, slightly on the radial side of the anterior wrist, at the same level as the area indicated in Fig. 18. This image shows only the radial side.

Anatomical Landmarks: The flexor carpi radialis tendon over the scaphoid bone.

Surrounding Structures: The median nerve is situated in the superficial space, between the third and fourth tendons of the flexor digitorum superficialis.

Additional Observation: This image shows the proximal carpal tunnel as well as the flexor retinaculum.

Fig. 20 Median Nerve / Distal Carpal Tunnel / Trapezium / Abductor Pollicis Brevis Muscle / Superficial Head of Flexor Pollicis Brevis Muscle

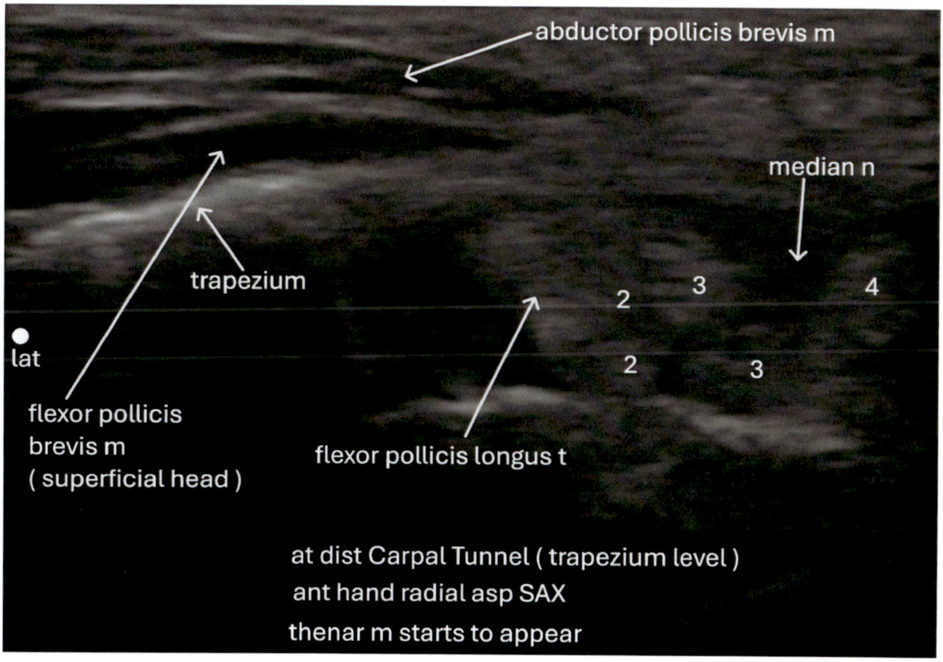

Probe Position: The probe is placed transversely, slightly on the radial side of the anterior wrist, just distal to the area indicated in Fig. 10.

Anatomical Landmark: The trapezium bone.

Surrounding Structures: The median nerve is located between the third and fourth tendons of the flexor digitorum superficialis. At this level, two thenar muscles are visualized: the superficial head of the flexor pollicis brevis muscle is situated on the trapezium bone, and just superficial to this muscle, the abductor pollicis brevis muscle can be seen.

Additional Observations: This image shows the radial aspect of the distal Carpal Tunnel. This level and more distally, the thenar muscles can be visualized.

Fig. 21 Median Nerve / Base of 1st Metacarpal / Abductor Pollicis Brevis Muscle / Superficial Head of Flexor Pollicis Brevis Muscle

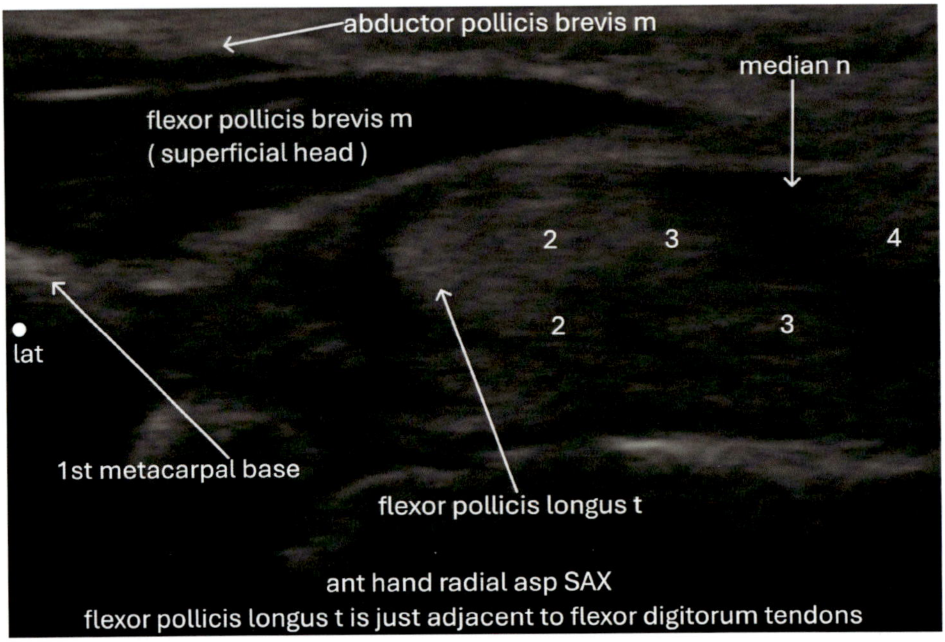

Probe Position: The probe is placed transversely, slightly on the radial side of the anterior hand, just distal to the area indicated in Fig. 20.

Anatomical Landmark: The base of the 1st metacarpal.

Surrounding Structures: The median nerve is located between the third and fourth tendons of the flexor digitorum superficialis. At this level, two thenar muscles are visualized: the superficial head of the flexor pollicis brevis muscle and the abductor pollicis brevis muscle, which is now situated superficial and more lateral compared to the former muscle.

Additional Observation: The flexor pollicis longus tendon is still just adjacent to the flexor digitorum superficialis and profundus tendons for the second digit.

Fig. 22 Recurrent Motor Branch of Median Nerve / Median Nerve / Proximal Metacarpals / Opponens Pollicis Muscle / Deep Head of Flexor Pollicis Brevis Muscle

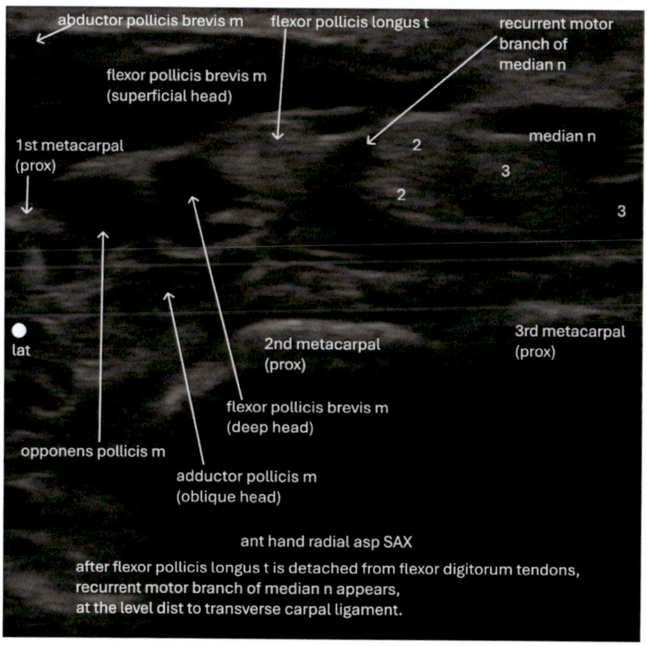

Probe Position: The probe is placed transversely, slightly on the radial side of the anterior hand, just distal to the area indicated in Fig. 21.

Anatomical Landmarks: The proximal level of the 3rd metacarpal and the flexor pollicis longus tendon.

Surrounding Structures: The median nerve is located between the third and fourth tendons of the flexor digitorum superficialis. At this level, the recurrent motor branch of the median nerve is visualized just deep to the superficial head of the flexor pollicis brevis, located between the tendon of the flexor pollicis longus and the tendons of the flexor digitorum superficialis and profundus to the index finger. In this image, the recurrent motor branch is observed distal to its origin. Additionally, two other thenar muscles are visible here: the deep head of the flexor pollicis brevis muscle, situated just lateral to the flexor pollicis longus tendon, and the opponens pollicis muscle, found between the deep head of the flexor pollicis brevis muscle and the proximal level of the 1st metacarpal.

Additional Observation: The flexor pollicis longus tendon is now separated from the second tendons of the flexor digitorum superficialis and profundus.

Fig. 23 Recurrent Motor Branch of Median Nerve / Common Palmar Digital Nerves of Median Nerve / Mid-Shaft Metacarpals / Oblique and Transverse Heads of Adductor Pollicis Muscle

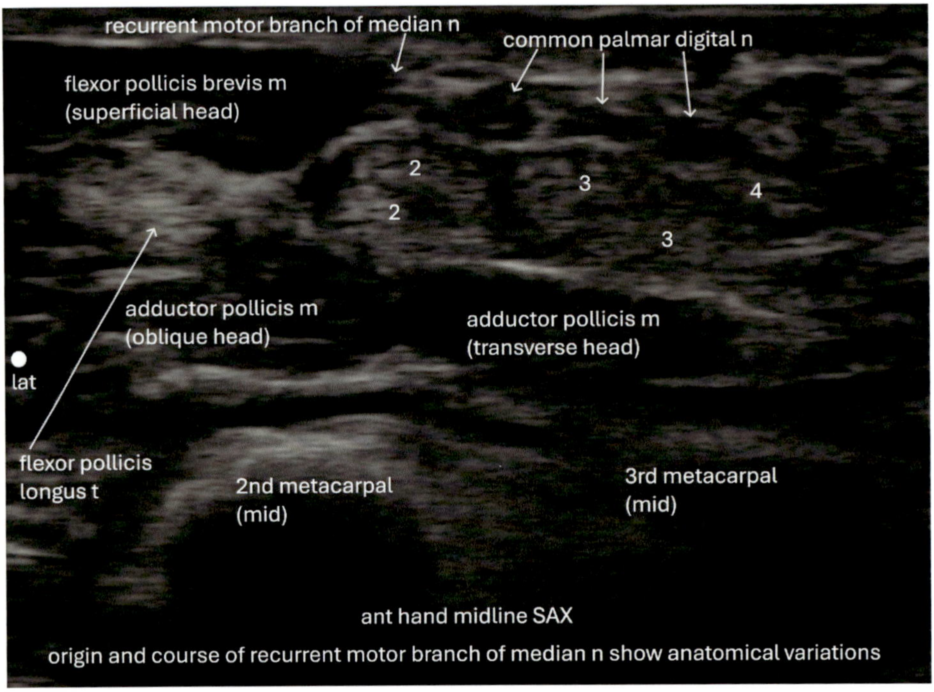

Probe Position: The probe is placed transversely on the midline of the anterior hand, just distal to the area indicated in Fig. 22.

Anatomical Landmark: The mid-shaft of the 3rd metacarpal.

Surrounding Structures: Distal to the carpal tunnel, the median nerve divides into three common palmar digital nerves, which further branch into proper palmar digital nerves. The recurrent motor branch of the median nerve typically curves superficially along the edge of the superficial head of the flexor pollicis brevis, running between the abductor pollicis brevis and the superficial head of the flexor pollicis brevis. Its origin and course may vary anatomically.

Additional Observations: In the deep layer, two other thenar muscles are visible here: the oblique and transverse heads of the adductor pollicis muscle.

Fig. 24 Thenar Muscles / Mid-Shaft Metacarpals / 1st Dorsal Interosseous Muscle

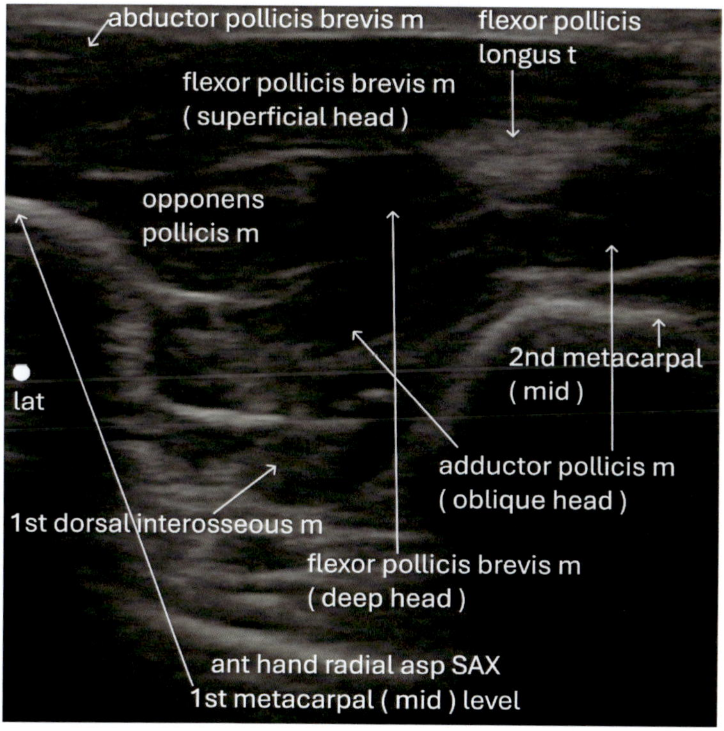

Probe Position: The probe is placed transversely on the radial side of the anterior hand, at the same level as the area indicated in Fig. 23.

Anatomical Landmarks: The mid-shaft of the 1st and 2nd metacarpals.

Visualized Structures: The thenar muscles visible are:

- Superficial layer: Abductor pollicis brevis and the superficial head of the flexor pollicis brevis.
- Middle layer: Opponens pollicis, the flexor pollicis longus tendon, and the deep head of the flexor pollicis brevis. (The deep head of the flexor pollicis brevis appears between the opponens pollicis and the flexor pollicis longus tendon, but it's actually situated slightly deep and medial to the opponens pollicis, and also passes deep to the flexor pollicis longus tendon.)
- Deep layer: Oblique head of the adductor pollicis.

Other Structure: Deeper to the oblique head of the adductor pollicis muscle, the 1st dorsal interosseous muscle can be seen.

Fig. 25 Thenar Muscles / 1st Distal Metacarpal / Mid-Shaft of 2nd Metacarpal / 1st Dorsal Interosseous Muscle

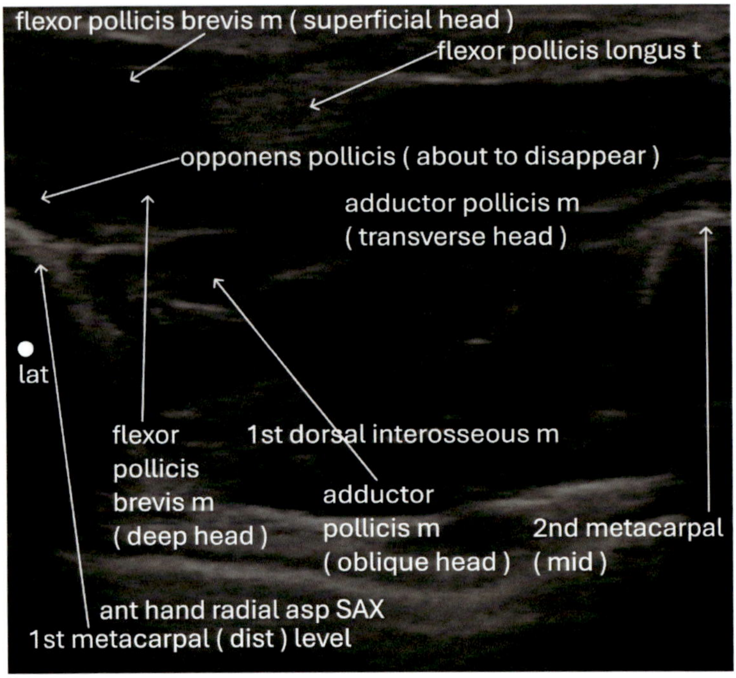

Probe Position: The probe is placed transversely on the radial side of the anterior hand, just distal to the area indicated in Fig. 24.

Anatomical Landmarks: The distal level of the 1st metacarpal and the mid-shaft of the 2nd metacarpal.

Visualized Structures: The thenar muscles visible are:

- Towards the lateral sesamoid bone of the thumb: the abductor pollicis brevis, the superficial head of the flexor pollicis brevis, and the deep head of the flexor pollicis brevis.
- Towards the medial sesamoid bone of the thumb: the oblique and transverse heads of the adductor pollicis.
- The opponens pollicis moves out of view for its insertion to the distal level of the 1st metacarpal.

Other Structure: Deeper to the transverse head of the adductor pollicis muscle, the 1st dorsal interosseous muscle can be seen.

Fig. 26 Thenar Muscle / 1st Distal Metacarpal / Mid-Shaft of 2nd Metacarpal / 1st Dorsal Interosseous Muscle

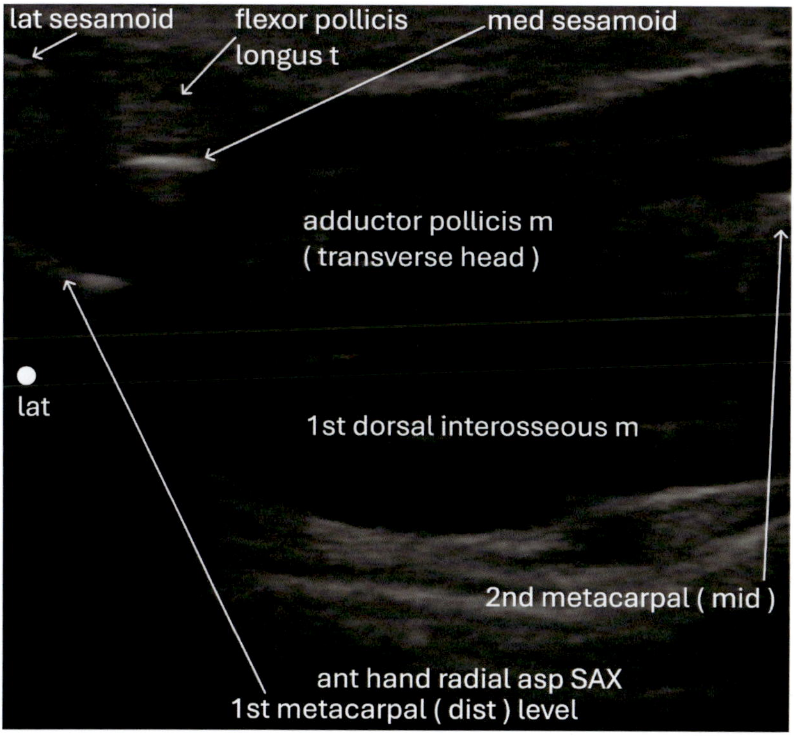

Probe Position: The probe is placed transversely on the radial side of the anterior hand, just distal to the area indicated in Fig. 25.

Anatomical Landmarks: The lateral and medial sesamoid bones of the thumb.

Visualized Structures: The two muscles visible here are the transverse head of the adductor pollicis muscle and the first dorsal interosseous muscle.

Other Structures: The flexor pollicis longus tendon can be seen between the lateral and medial sesamoid bones, over the distal level of the first metacarpal.

Fig. 27 Thenar Muscle / 1st Proximal Phalanx / 2nd Distal Metacarpal / 1st Lumbrical Muscle / 1st Dorsal Interosseous Muscle

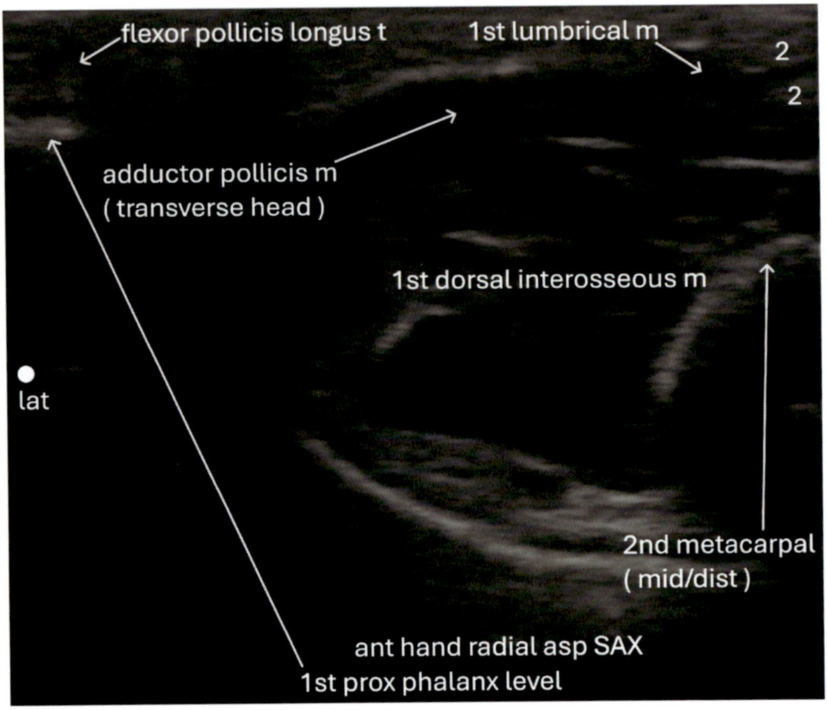

Probe Position: The probe is placed transversely on the radial side of the anterior hand, just distal to the area indicated in Fig. 26.

Anatomical Landmarks: The flexor pollicis longus tendon over the proximal phalanx of the thumb.

Visualized Structures: The transverse head of the adductor pollicis muscle, which is reduced in size here, is the only thenar muscle remaining visible (although, strictly speaking, the adductor pollicis muscle is not a thenar muscle). The first dorsal interosseous muscle occupies the majority of the space just lateral to the second metacarpal.

Other Structure: The first lumbrical muscle can be seen just lateral to the flexor digitorum superficialis and profundus tendons for the second digit.

Fig. 28 1st Proximal Phalanx / 2nd Distal Metacarpal / 1st Lumbrical Muscle / 1st Dorsal Interosseous Muscle

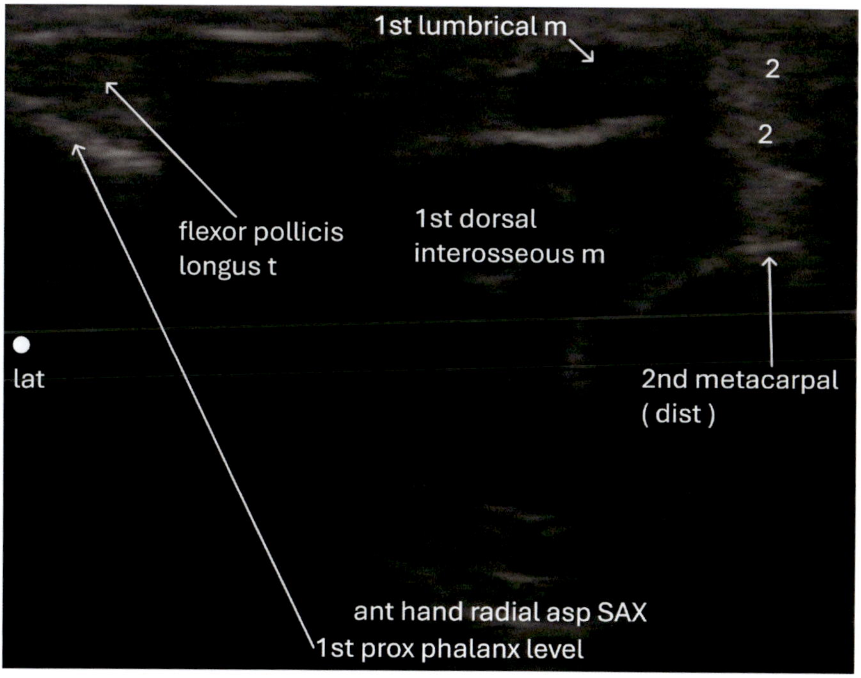

Probe Position: The probe is placed transversely on the radial side of the anterior hand, just distal to the area indicated in Fig. 27.

Anatomical Landmark: The distal level of the second metacarpal.

Visualized Structures: After the transverse head of the adductor pollicis muscle moves out of view, no more thenar muscle is seen. Here are the two muscles visible: the first lumbrical muscle superficially, and deep to that, the first dorsal interosseous muscle which can be seen just lateral to the distal level of the second metacarpal.

Additional Observation: The first lumbrical muscle can be seen just lateral to the tendons for the second digit of the flexor digitorum superficialis and profundus muscles.

SECTION 3

Fig. 1 Superficial Branch of Radial Nerve / Deep Branch of Radial Nerve / Articular Cartilage of Anterior Elbow / Brachialis Muscle / Brachioradialis Muscle

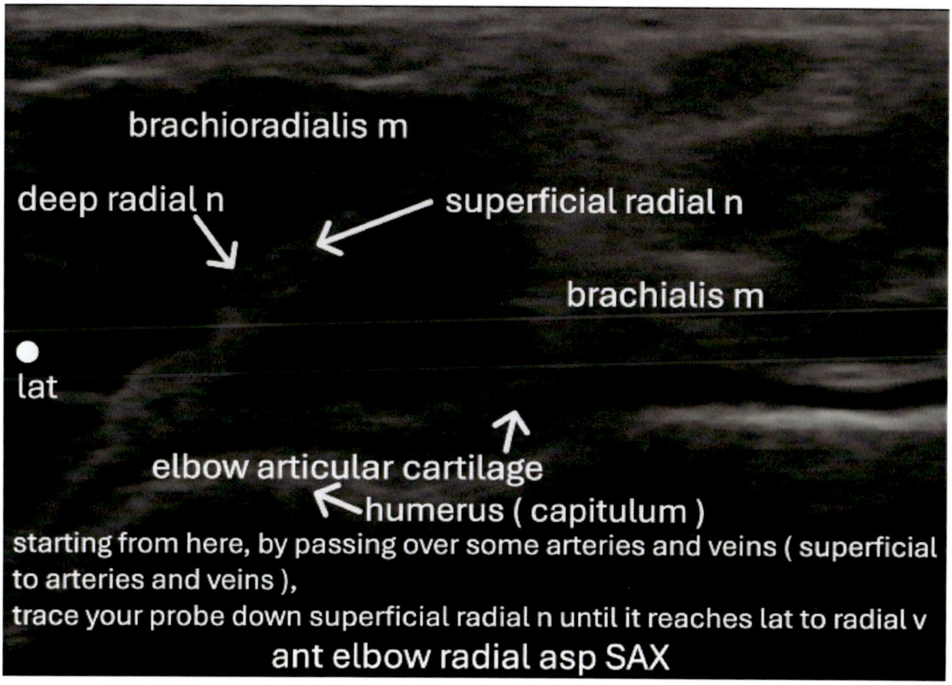

Probe Position: The probe is placed transversely (with its axis perpendicular to the arm) immediately proximal to the radial side of the elbow crease.

Anatomical Landmark: The anterior elbow articular cartilage at the capitulum of the humerus.

Surrounding Structures: The superficial branch of the radial nerve is located between the brachialis and brachioradialis muscles, and just superficial to the deep branch of the radial nerve, which will become the posterior interosseous nerve further distally.

Additional Observation: Scanning from this position distally, the superficial branch of the radial nerve is viewed as passing just superficial to the arteries and veins until it reaches the area just lateral to the radial vein and superficial to the supinator muscle.

Fig. 2 Superficial Branch of Radial Nerve / Radial Artery / Radial Vein / Supinator Muscle / Humeral Head of Pronator Teres Muscle

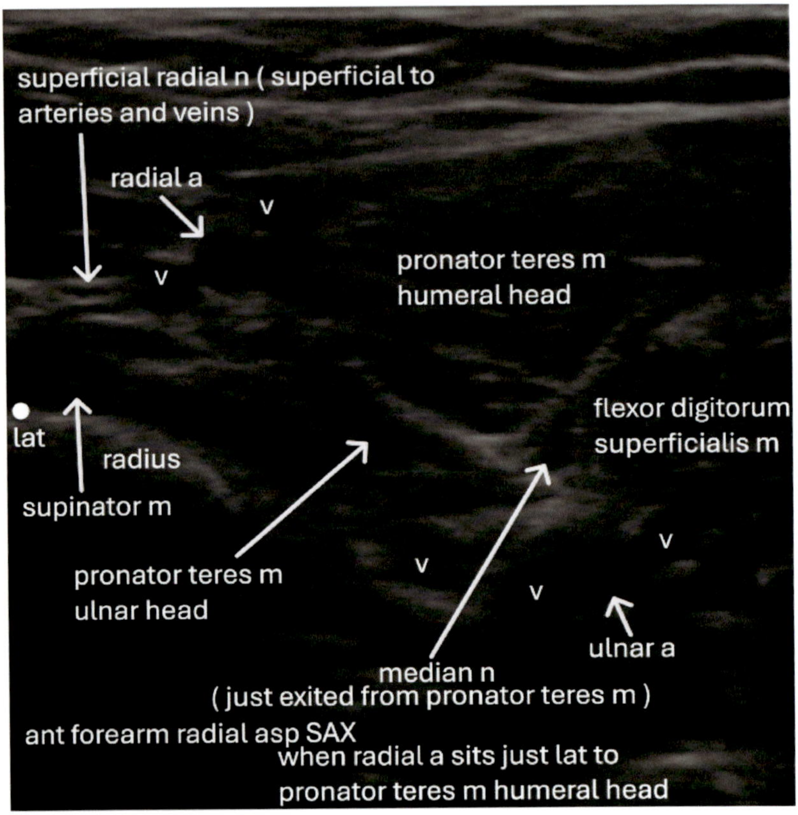

Probe Position: The probe is placed transversely, slightly on the radial side of the proximal forearm, distal to the location depicted in Fig. 1.

Anatomical Landmarks: The radial artery, which is found at the lateral edge of the humeral head of the pronator teres muscle.

Surrounding Structures: The superficial branch of the radial nerve is located just lateral to the radial vein and superficial to the supinator muscle.

Additional Observation: At this level, the median nerve has just exited the space between the two heads of the pronator teres muscle.

Fig. 3 Superficial Branch of Radial Nerve / Radial Artery / Radial Vein / Supinator Muscle / Humeral Head of Pronator Teres Muscle

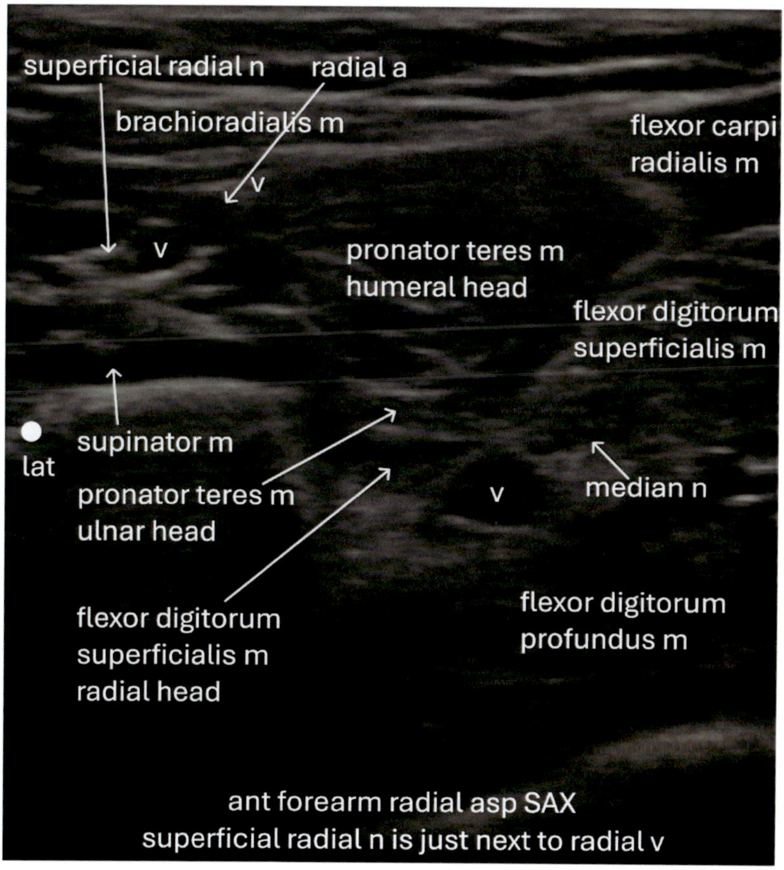

Probe Position: The probe is placed transversely, slightly on the radial side of the proximal forearm, immediately distal to the location shown in Fig. 2.

Anatomical Landmarks: The radial artery, which is found at the lateral edge of the humeral head of the pronator teres muscle.

Surrounding Structures: The superficial branch of the radial nerve is located just lateral to the radial vein and superficial to the supinator muscle.

Additional Observation: At this level, the radial head of the flexor digitorum superficialis muscle appears.

Fig. 4 Superficial Branch of Radial Nerve / Radial Artery / Radial Vein / Supinator Muscle / Humeral Head of Pronator Teres Muscle

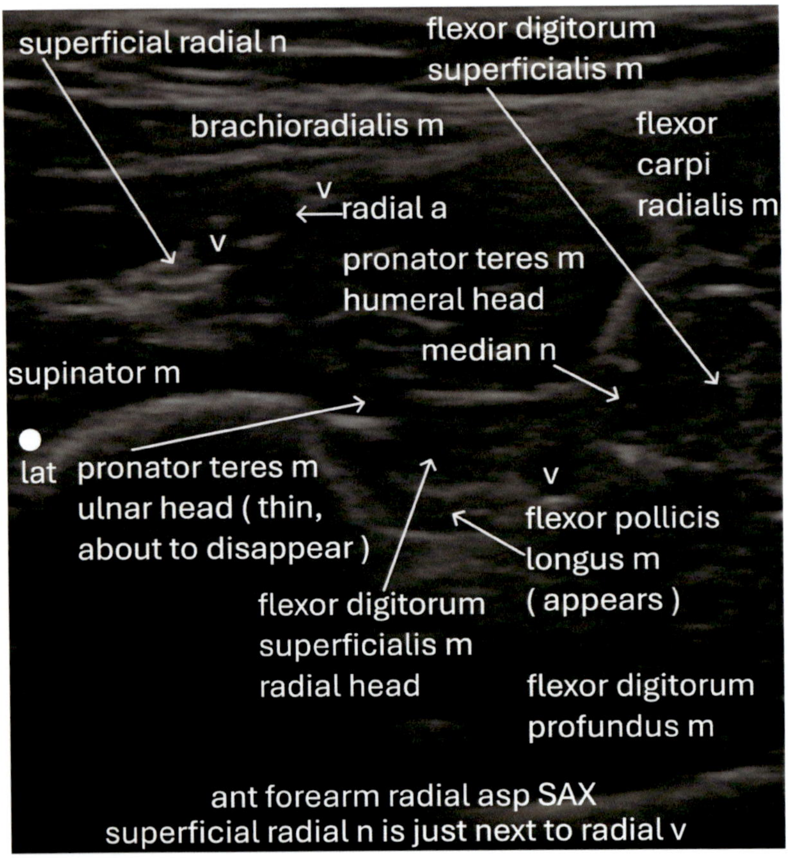

Probe Position: The probe is placed transversely, slightly on the radial side of the proximal forearm, immediately distal to the location shown in Fig. 3.

Anatomical Landmarks: The radial artery, which is found at the lateral edge of the humeral head of the pronator teres muscle.

Surrounding Structures: The superficial branch of the radial nerve is located just lateral to the radial vein and superficial to the supinator muscle.

Additional Observation: At this level, the flexor pollicis longus muscle appears.

Fig. 5 Superficial Branch of Radial Nerve / Radial Artery / Radial Vein / Supinator Muscle / Humeral Head of Pronator Teres Muscle

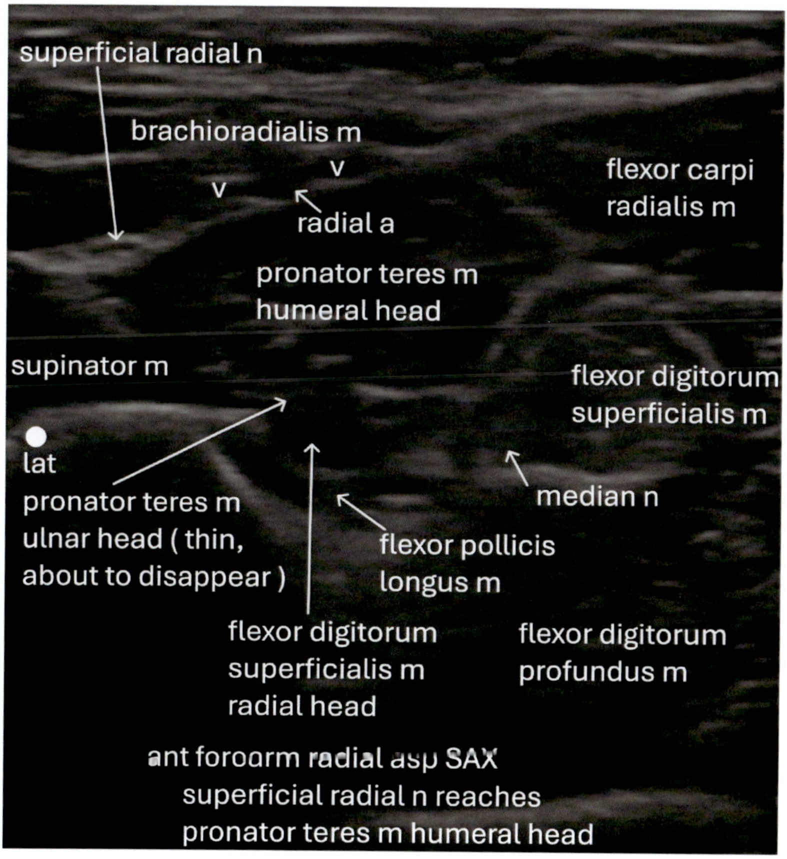

Probe Position: The probe is placed transversely, slightly on the radial side of the mid-forearm, immediately distal to the location shown in Fig. 4.

Anatomical Landmarks: The radial artery, which is located on the superficial surface of the mid-portion of the humeral head of the pronator teres muscle.

Surrounding Structure: The superficial branch of the radial nerve is found on the superficial surface of the lateral edge of the humeral head of the pronator teres muscle.

Additional Observation: At this level, the superficial branch of the radial nerve and the radial vein are separated.

Fig. 6 Superficial Branch of Radial Nerve / Brachioradialis Muscle / Humeral Head of Pronator Teres Muscle / Radial Artery / Flexor Carpi Radialis Muscle

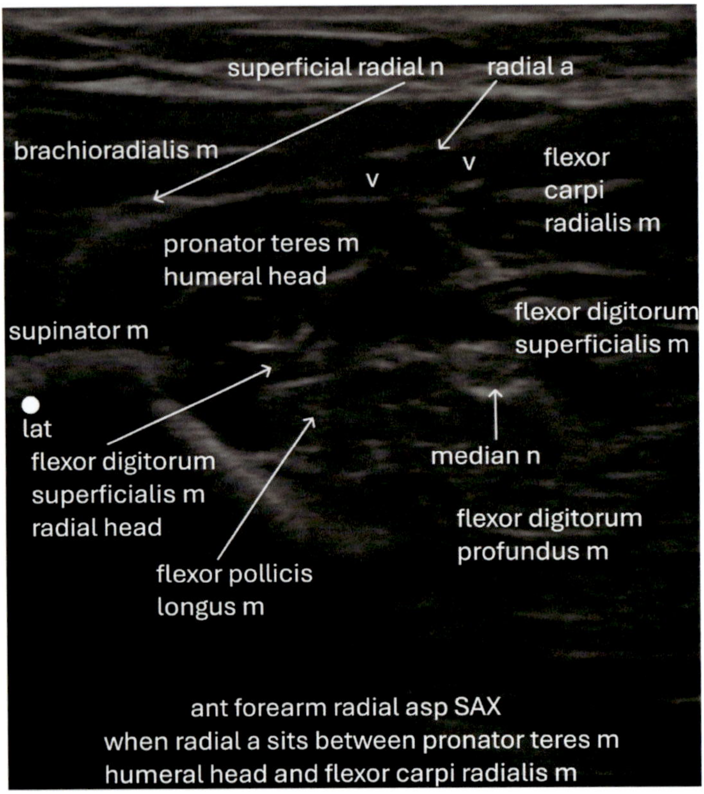

Probe Position: The probe is placed transversely, slightly on the radial side of the mid-forearm, immediately distal to the location shown in Fig. 5.

Anatomical Landmarks: The radial artery, which lies between the humeral head of the pronator teres muscle and the flexor carpi radialis muscle.

Surrounding Structure: The superficial branch of the radial nerve is found on the superficial surface of the lateral part of the humeral head of the pronator teres muscle.

Additional Observation: The superficial branch of the radial nerve is located between the brachioradialis muscle and the humeral head of the pronator teres muscle.

Fig. 7 Superficial Branch of Radial Nerve / Brachioradialis Muscle / Humeral Head of Pronator Teres Muscle / Radial Artery / Flexor Carpi Radialis Muscle

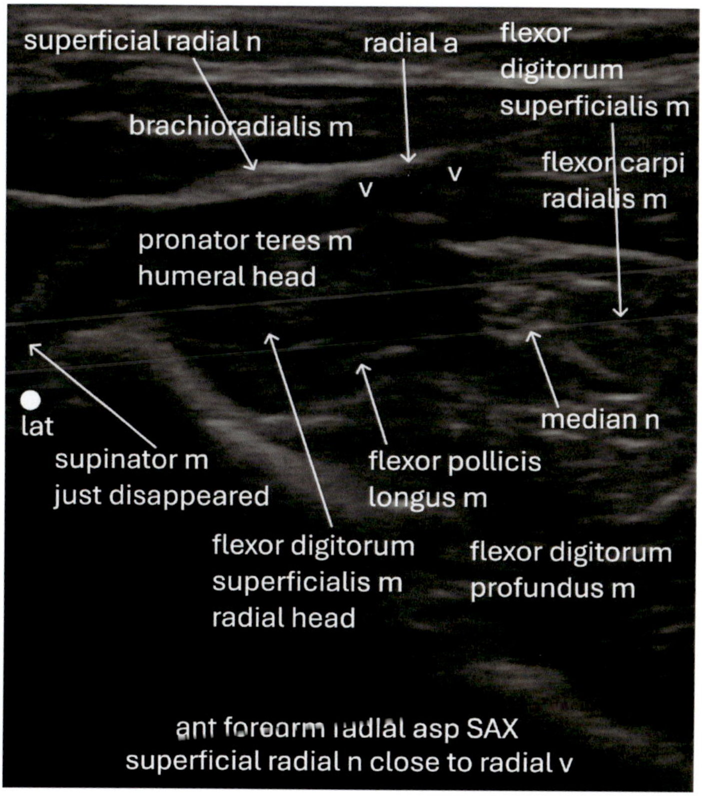

Probe Position: The probe is placed transversely, slightly on the radial side of the mid-forearm, immediately distal to the location shown in Fig. 6.

Anatomical Landmarks: The radial artery, which lies between the humeral head of the pronator teres muscle and the flexor carpi radialis muscle.

Surrounding Structure: The superficial branch of the radial nerve is found on the superficial surface of the mid-portion of the humeral head of the pronator teres muscle.

Additional Observations: The superficial branch of the radial nerve is located between the brachioradialis muscle and the humeral head of the pronator teres muscle. Additionally, the supinator muscle is no longer visible.

Fig. 8 Superficial Branch of Radial Nerve / Brachioradialis Muscle / Humeral Head of Pronator Teres Muscle / Radial Artery / Radial Vein / Flexor Carpi Radialis Muscle

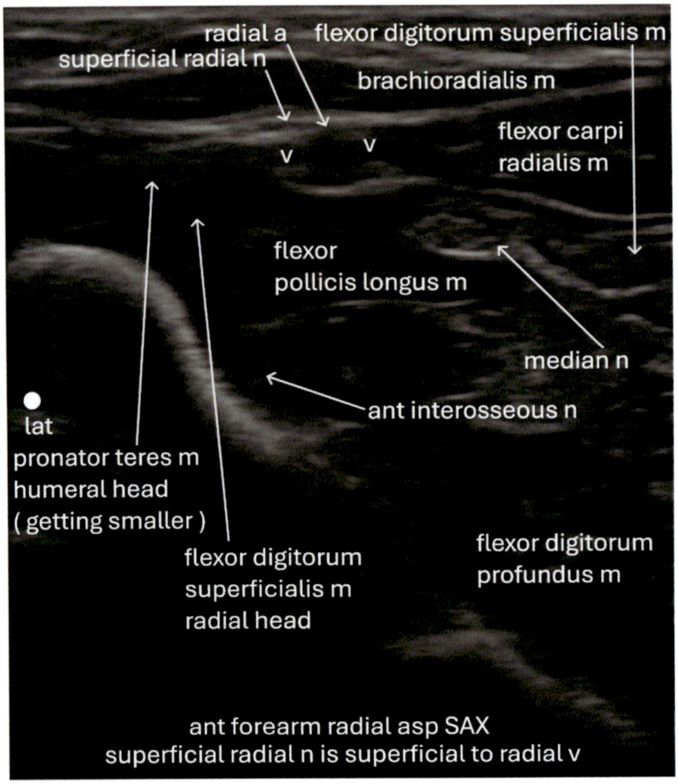

Probe Position: The probe is placed transversely, slightly on the radial side of the mid-forearm, immediately distal to the location shown in Fig. 7.

Anatomical Landmarks: The radial artery, which lies between the humeral head of the pronator teres muscle and the flexor carpi radialis muscle.

Surrounding Structure: The superficial branch of the radial nerve is found just superficial to the radial vein.

Additional Observations: The superficial branch of the radial nerve is located just deep to the brachioradialis muscle. Additionally, the humeral head of the pronator teres muscle has decreased in size at this level.

Fig. 9 Superficial Branch of Radial Nerve / Brachioradialis Muscle / Humeral Head of Pronator Teres Muscle / Radial Artery / Radial Vein / Flexor Carpi Radialis Muscle

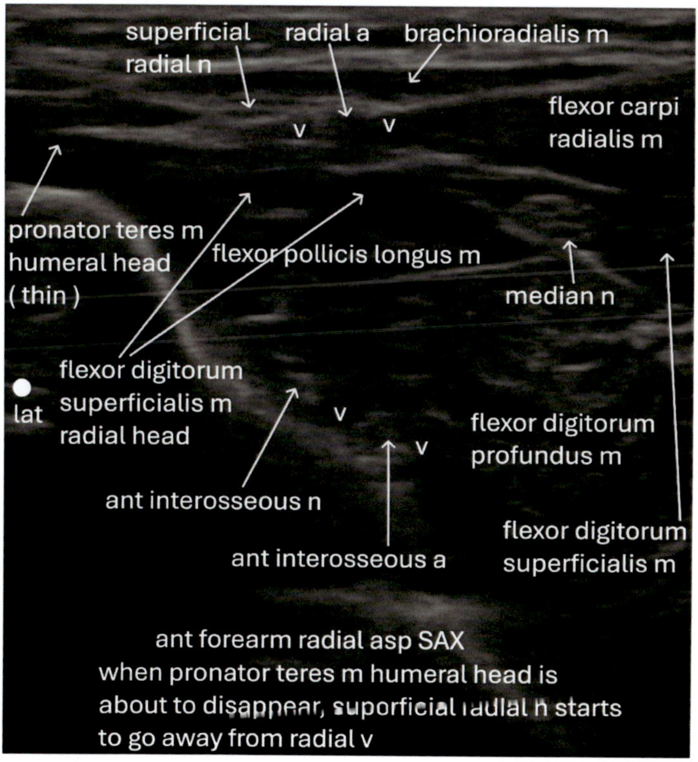

Probe Position: The probe is placed transversely, slightly on the radial side of the mid-forearm, immediately distal to the location shown in Fig. 8.

Anatomical Landmarks: The radial artery, which lies between the humeral head of the pronator teres muscle and the flexor carpi radialis muscle.

Surrounding Structure: The superficial branch of the radial nerve is found just superficial and lateral to the radial vein.

Additional Observations: The superficial branch of the radial nerve is located just deep to the brachioradialis muscle. Additionally, the humeral head of the pronator teres muscle is hardly visible at this level.

Fig. 10 Superficial Branch of Radial Nerve / Brachioradialis Muscle / Extensor Carpi Radialis Longus and Brevis Muscles

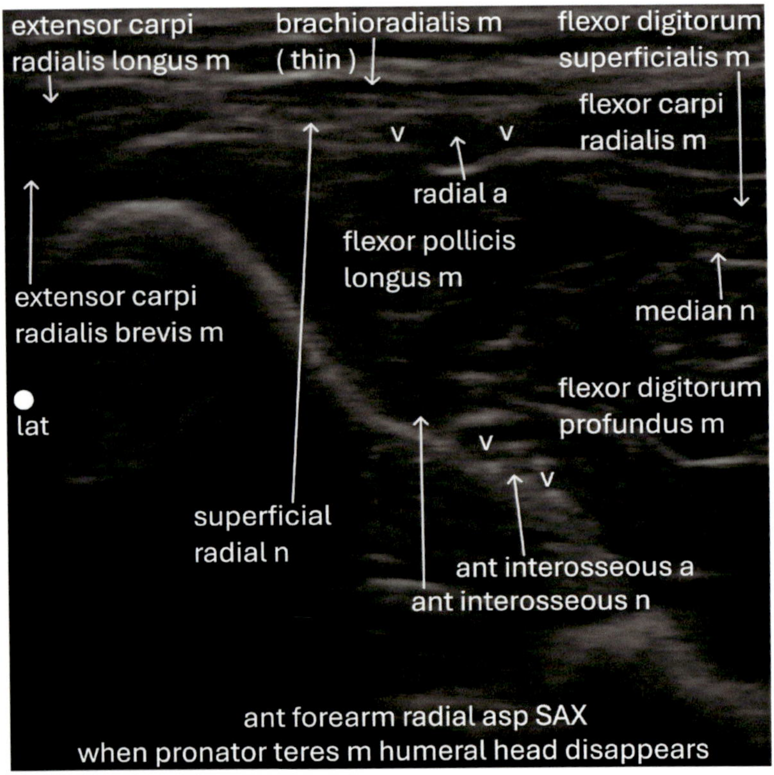

Probe Position: The probe is placed transversely, slightly on the radial side of the mid-forearm, immediately distal to the location shown in Fig. 9.

Anatomical Landmarks: The radial artery and veins, which lie just lateral to the flexor carpi radialis muscle.

Surrounding Structure: The superficial branch of the radial nerve is found just superficial and lateral to the radial vein.

Additional Observations: The superficial branch of the radial nerve is located just deep to the brachioradialis muscle, which is very thin at this level. The humeral head of the pronator teres muscle is no longer visible. The radial head of the flexor digitorum superficialis muscle will join the humeroulnar head medially. Additionally, the extensor carpi radialis longus and brevis muscles are visible on the lateral aspect of the radius.

Fig. 11 Superficial Branch of Radial Nerve / Musculotendinous Junction of Brachioradialis / Extensor Carpi Radialis Longus and Brevis Muscles

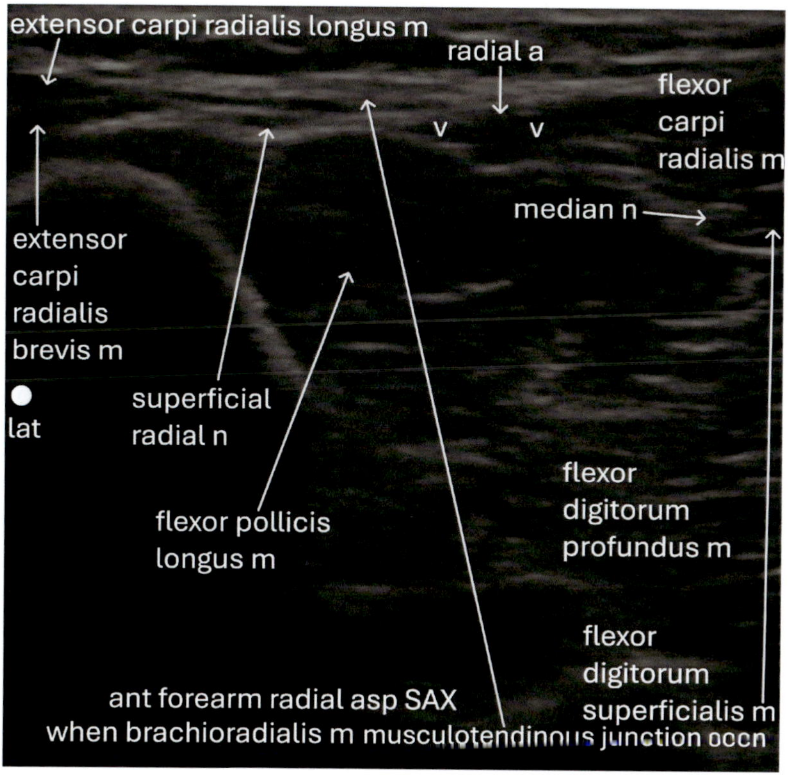

Probe Position: The probe is placed transversely, slightly on the radial side of the distal forearm, immediately distal to the location shown in Fig. 10.

Anatomical Landmarks: The radial artery and veins, which lie just lateral to the flexor carpi radialis muscle.

Surrounding Structure: The superficial branch of the radial nerve is visible deep to the musculotendinous junction of the brachioradialis muscle.

Additional Observations: The extensor carpi radialis longus and brevis muscles are visible on the lateral aspect of the radius.

Fig. 12 Superficial Branch of Radial Nerve / Tendons of Brachioradialis and Extensor Carpi Radialis Longus Muscles

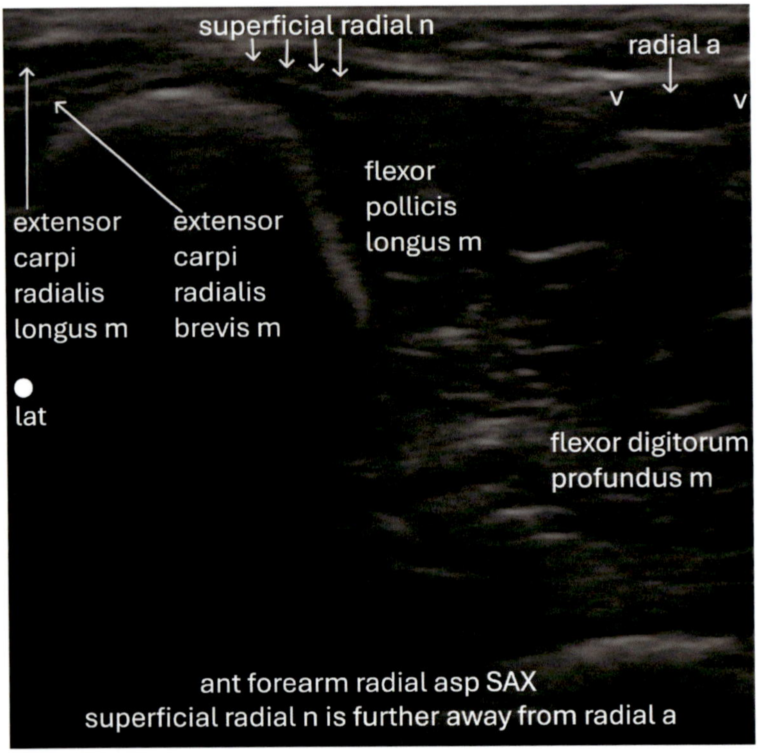

Probe Position: The probe is placed transversely on the radial side of the distal forearm, immediately distal to the location shown in Fig. 11.

Anatomical Landmarks: The radius and the flexor pollicis longus muscle.

Surrounding Structures: The superficial radial nerve is about to pierce the deep fascia to emerge superficially, positioned between the tendons of the brachioradialis and extensor carpi radialis longus in the distal forearm.

Additional Observations: At this level, the superficial branch of the radial nerve is further away from the radial vein. Additionally, the musculotendinous junctions of the extensor carpi radialis longus and brevis muscles are visible on the anterior aspect of the radius.

Fig. 13 Superficial Branch of Radial Nerve / Tendons of Brachioradialis and Extensor Carpi Radialis Longus Muscles

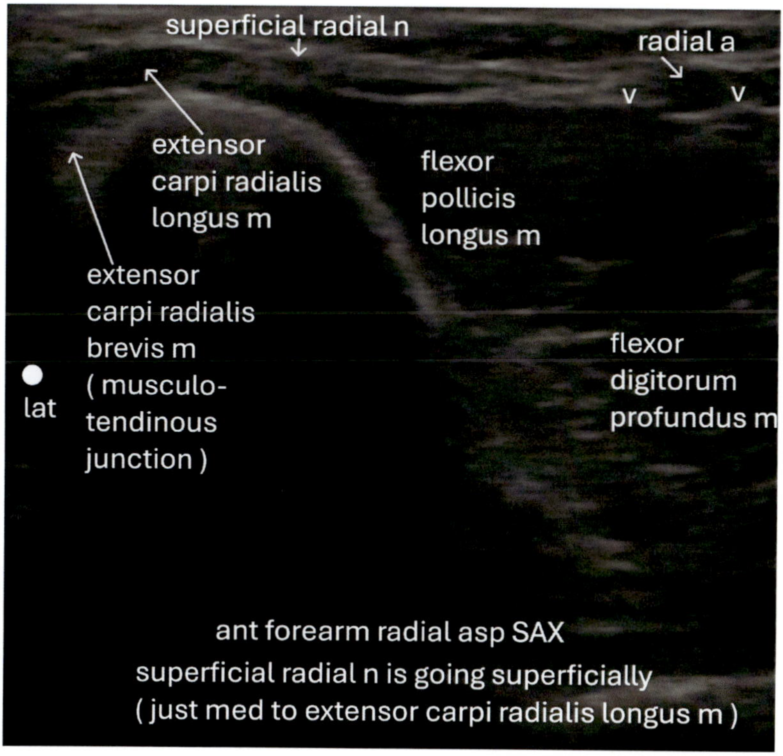

Probe Position: The probe is placed transversely on the radial side of the distal forearm, immediately distal to the location shown in Fig. 12.

Anatomical Landmarks: The space between the tendons of the brachioradialis and extensor carpi radialis longus muscles.

Surrounding Structures: The superficial branch of the radial nerve emerges superficially to the deep fascia, situated between the tendons of the brachioradialis and extensor carpi radialis longus muscles.

Additional Observations: The musculotendinous junctions of the extensor carpi radialis longus and brevis muscles are visible on the anterior aspect of the radius.

Fig. 14 Medial and Lateral Branches of Superficial Radial Nerve / Volar Branch of Lateral Antebrachial Cutaneous Nerve

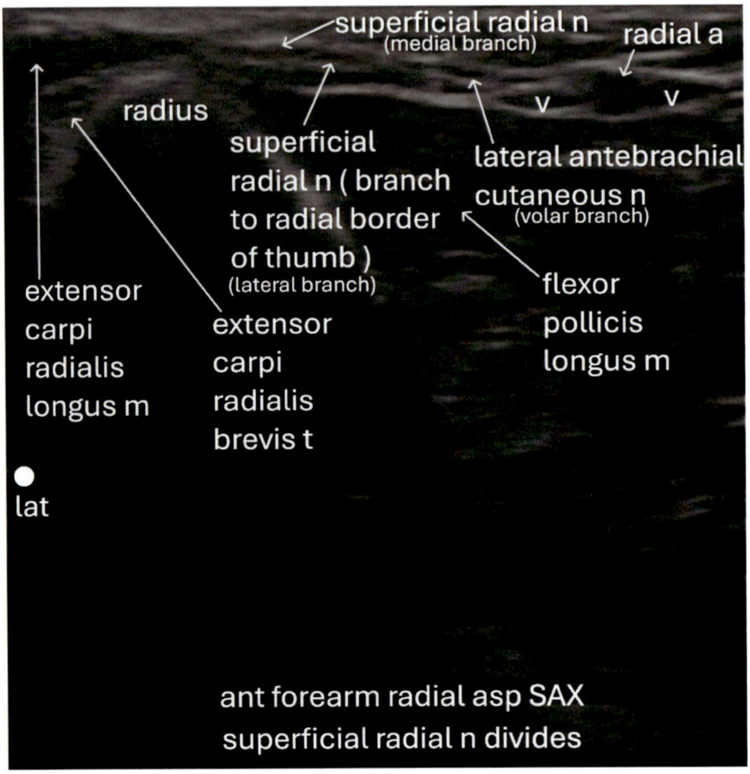

Probe Position: The probe is placed transversely on the radial side of the distal forearm, immediately distal to the location shown in Fig. 13.

Anatomical Landmark: The tendon of the extensor carpi radialis longus muscle.

Surrounding Structures: The superficial branch of the radial nerve divides into two branches: lateral and medial. The medial branch of the superficial radial nerve is the one that runs closer to the tendon of the extensor carpi radialis longus muscle.

Additional Observations: The volar branch of the lateral antebrachial cutaneous nerve can be seen just volar to the lateral branch of the superficial radial nerve. Additionally, the musculotendinous junctions of the extensor carpi radialis longus and brevis muscles are visible on the anterior aspect of the radius.

Fig. 15 Medial Branch of Superficial Radial Nerve / Abductor Pollicis Longus Muscle / Extensor Pollicis Brevis Muscle / Extensor Carpi Radialis Longus and Brevis Tendons

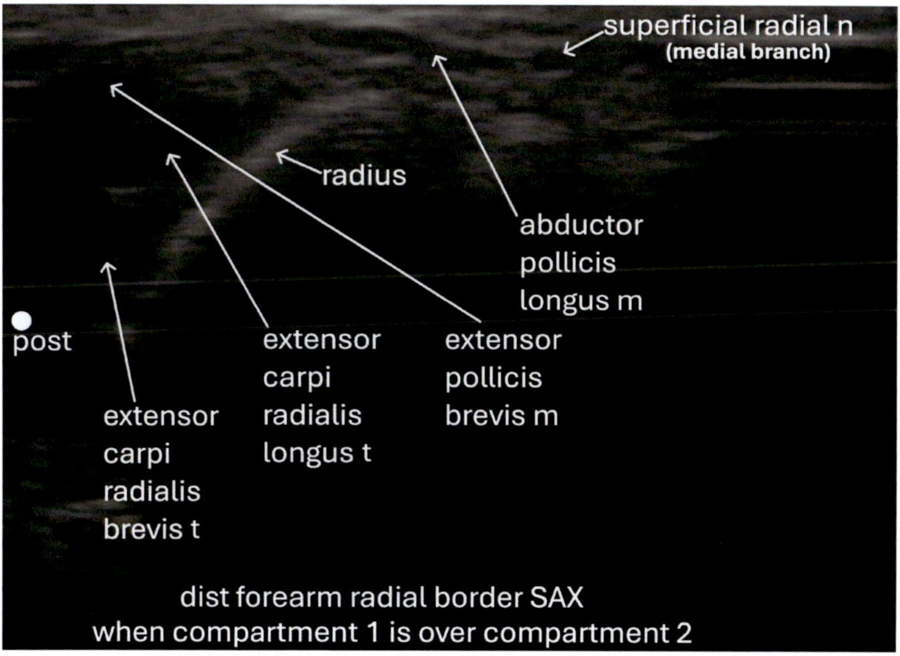

Probe Position: The probe is placed transversely on the radial border (between the anterior and posterior aspects) of the distal forearm, immediately distal to the location shown in Fig. 14.

Anatomical Landmark: The abductor pollicis longus muscle.

Surrounding Structures: The medial branch of the superficial radial nerve is about to course superficially over the top of the tendons of the abductor pollicis longus and extensor pollicis brevis muscles.

Additional Observation: The musculotendinous junctions of the abductor pollicis longus and extensor pollicis brevis muscles are crossing superficially over the tendons of the extensor carpi radialis longus and brevis muscles. (proximal intersection)

Fig. 16 Medial Branch of Superficial Radial Nerve / Abductor Pollicis Longus Tendon / Extensor Pollicis Brevis Tendon

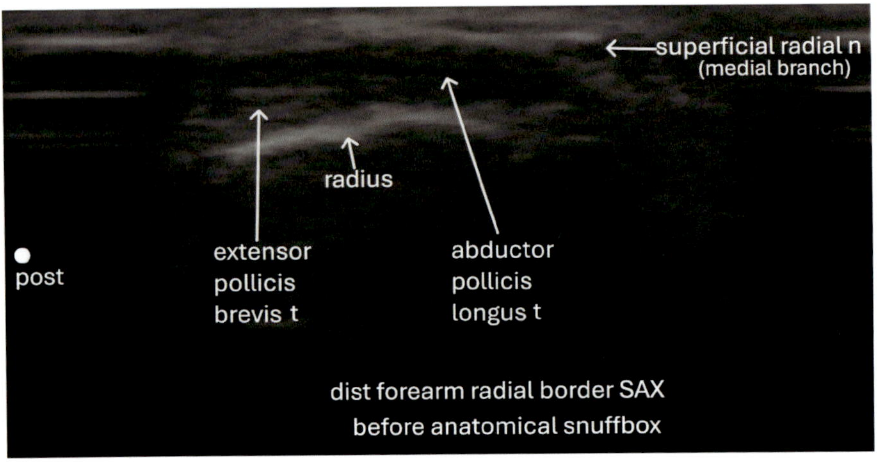

Probe Position: The probe is placed transversely on the radial border (between the anterior and posterior aspects) of the distal forearm, immediately distal to the location shown in Fig. 15.

Anatomical Landmark: The abductor pollicis longus tendon.

Surrounding Structure: In this view, the medial branch of the superficial radial nerve is at the starting position for crossing superficially over the abductor pollicis longus tendon.

Additional Observation: The tendons of the extensor carpi radialis longus and brevis muscles are not included in the left side of the field of view due to this probe position.

Fig. 17 Medial Branch of Superficial Radial Nerve / Abductor Pollicis Longus Tendon / Extensor Pollicis Brevis Tendon

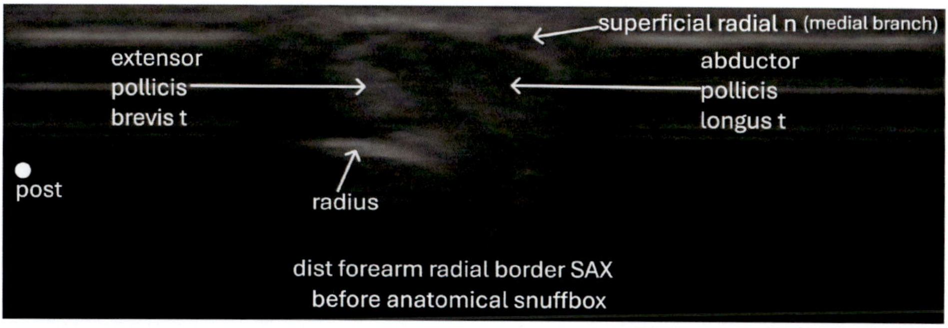

Probe Position: The probe is placed transversely on the radial border (between the anterior and posterior aspects) of the distal forearm, immediately distal to the location shown in Fig. 16.

Anatomical Landmark: The abductor pollicis longus tendon.

Surrounding Structure: In this view, the medial branch of the superficial radial nerve is crossing superficially over the abductor pollicis longus tendon.

Additional Observation: The first extensor compartment of the wrist, which contains the tendons of the abductor pollicis longus and extensor pollicis brevis, is located between the radius and the extensor retinaculum.

Fig. 18 Medial Branch of Superficial Radial Nerve / Abductor Pollicis Longus Tendon / Extensor Pollicis Brevis Tendon / Extensor Carpi Radialis Longus and Brevis Tendons

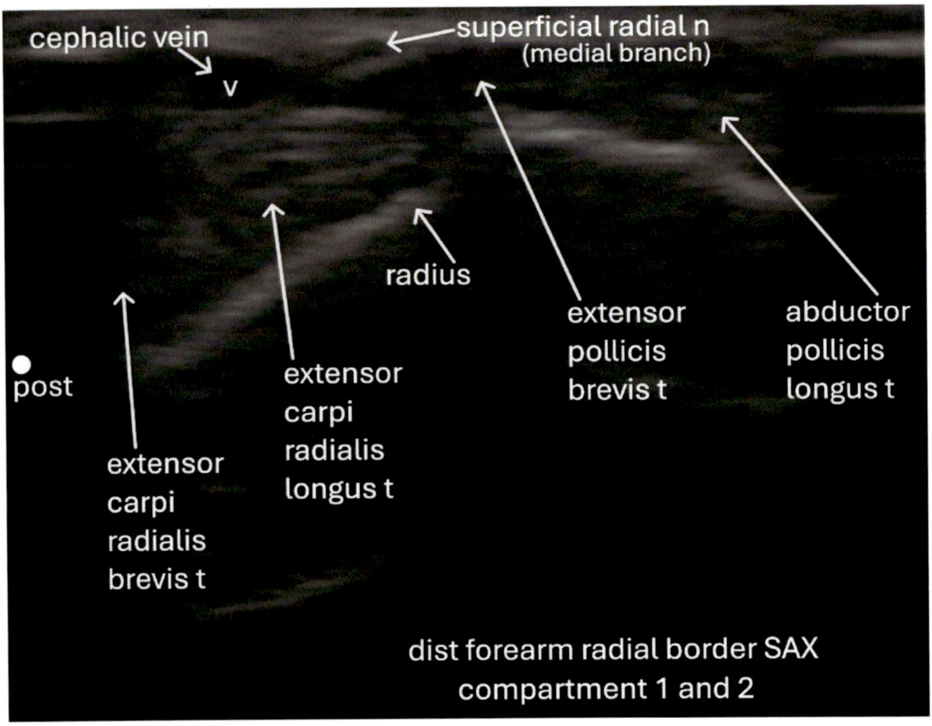

Probe Position: The probe is placed transversely on the radial border (between the anterior and posterior aspects) of the distal forearm, immediately distal to the location shown in Fig. 17.

Anatomical Landmark: The extensor pollicis brevis tendon.

Surrounding Structure: In this view, the medial branch of the superficial radial nerve is crossing superficially over the extensor pollicis brevis tendon.

Additional Observation: At this level, the second extensor compartment of the wrist, which contains the tendons of the extensor carpi radialis longus and brevis, comes back into view.

Fig. 19 Ulnar and Radial Branches of Medial Branch of Superficial Radial Nerve / Cephalic Vein / Extensor Pollicis Brevis Tendon

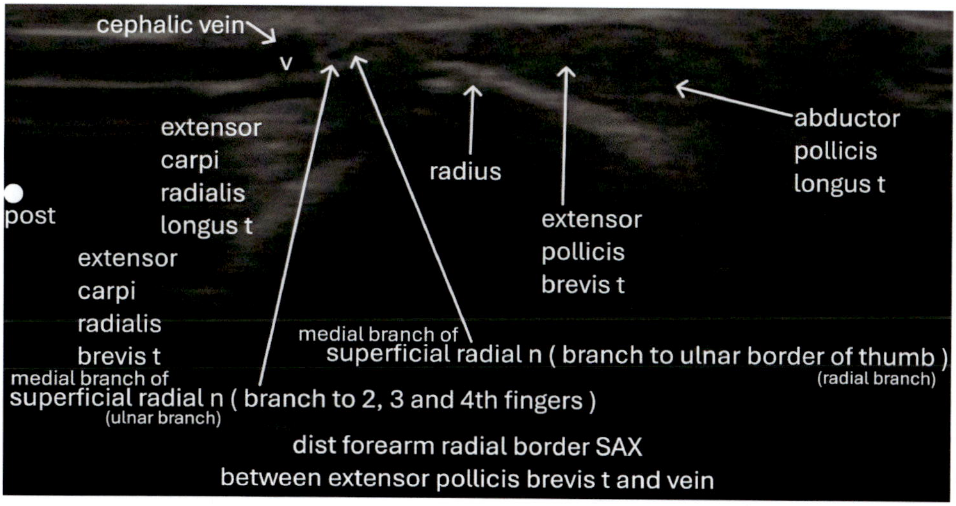

Probe Position: The probe is placed transversely on the radial border (between the anterior and posterior aspects) of the distal forearm, immediately distal to the location shown in Fig. 18.

Anatomical Landmarks: The space between the extensor pollicis brevis tendon and the cephalic vein.

Surrounding Structures: Immediately after crossing over the tendons of the first compartment, the medial branch of the superficial radial nerve divides into two branches on the radial side of the cephalic vein. (Anatomical variants are possible.) Of these two branches, the radial branch travels to the ulnar border of the thumb by crossing over the extensor pollicis longus tendon distally. The ulnar branch travels to the ulnar side of the cephalic vein to supply the rest of the superficial branch of the radial nerve's distribution.

Additional Observation: The extensor retinaculum of the extensor carpi radialis longus tendon is visible near the cephalic vein.

Fig. 20 Ulnar Branch of Medial Branch of Superficial Radial Nerve / Cephalic Vein / Extensor Retinaculum of the Second Compartment / Anatomical Snuffbox

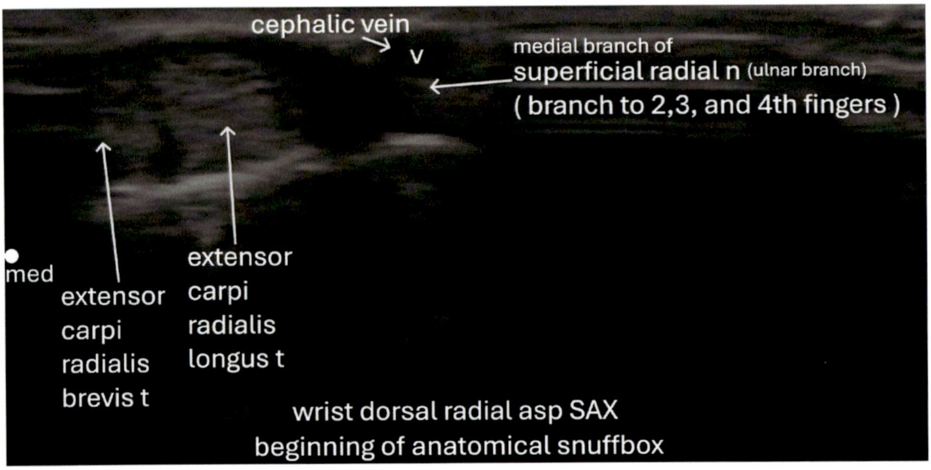

Probe Position: The probe is placed transversely on the dorsal-radial aspect of the wrist, just distal to the location shown in Fig. 19.

Anatomical Landmark: The proximal region of the anatomical snuffbox.

Surrounding Structure: The ulnar branch of the medial branch of the superficial radial nerve crosses underneath the cephalic vein. (Anatomical variants are possible.)

Additional Observation: The extensor retinaculum covering the second compartment is visible just ulnar (medial) to the cephalic vein.

Fig. 21 Ulnar Branch of Medial Branch of Superficial Radial Nerve / Cephalic Vein / Extensor Retinaculum of the Second Compartment / Anatomical Snuffbox

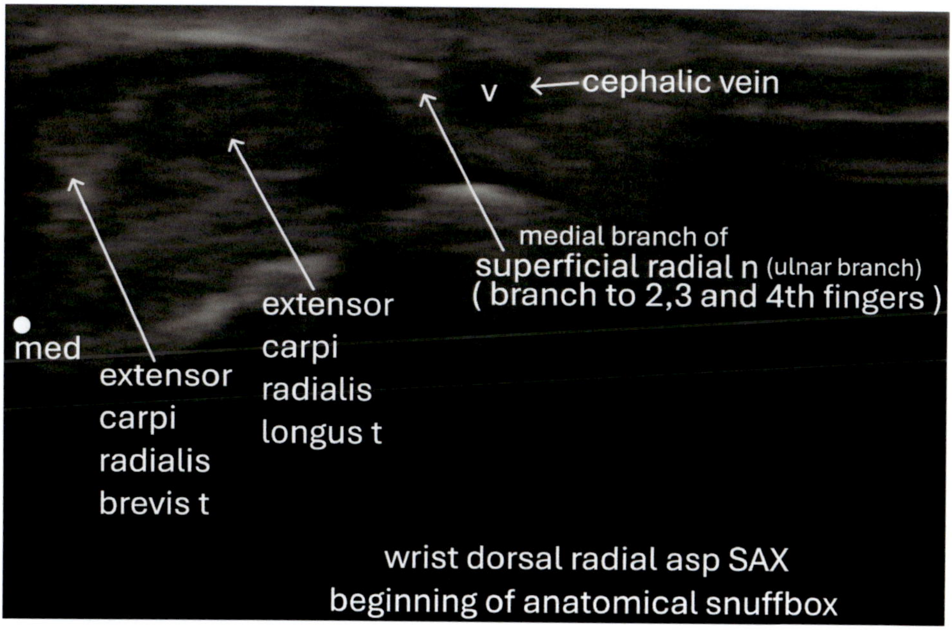

Probe Position: The probe is placed transversely on the dorsal-radial aspect of the wrist, just distal to the location shown in Fig. 20.

Anatomical Landmark: The proximal region of the anatomical snuffbox.

Surrounding Structures: The ulnar branch of the medial branch of the superficial radial nerve is situated between the cephalic vein and the extensor retinaculum, which covers the second compartment.

Additional Observation: The ulnar branch of the medial branch of the superficial radial nerve is now located on the ulnar side of the cephalic vein.

Fig. 22 Ulnar Branch of Medial Branch of Superficial Radial Nerve / Cephalic Vein / Extensor Pollicis Longus Tendon / Anatomical Snuffbox

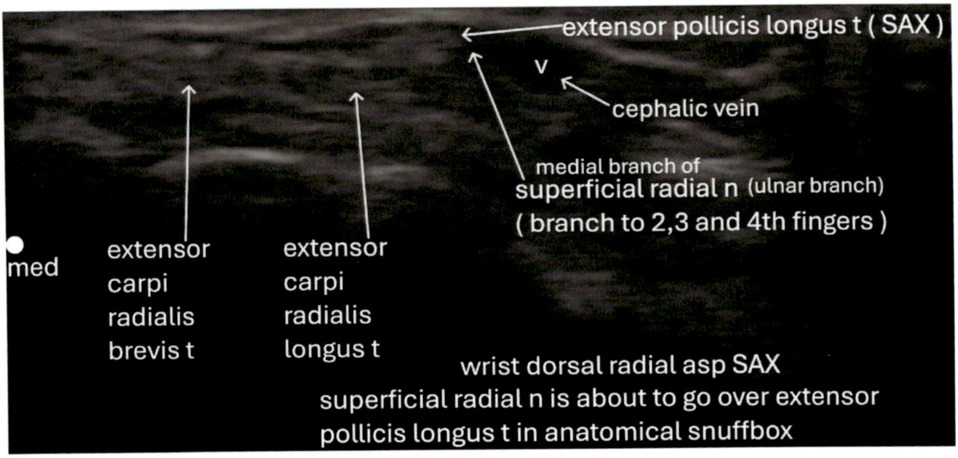

Probe Position: The probe is placed transversely on the dorsal-radial aspect of the wrist, just distal to the location shown in Fig. 21.

Anatomical Landmark: The middle region of the anatomical snuffbox.

Surrounding Structure: The ulnar branch of the medial branch of the superficial radial nerve is located on the radial side of the extensor pollicis longus tendon, which crosses superficially over the tendons of the second compartment at the distal intersection.

Additional Observation: The ulnar branch of the medial branch of the superficial radial nerve is about to cross the extensor pollicis longus tendon.

Fig. 23 Ulnar Branch of Medial Branch of Superficial Radial Nerve / Cephalic Vein / Extensor Pollicis Longus Tendon

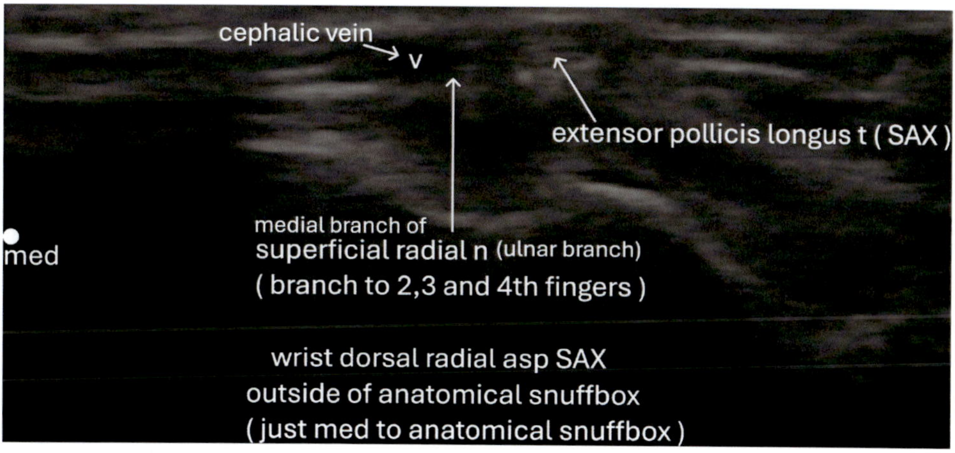

Probe Position: The probe is placed transversely on the dorsal-radial aspect of the wrist, just distal to the location shown in Fig. 22.

Anatomical Landmark: The region just medial (ulnar) to the extensor pollicis longus tendon (outside of the anatomical snuffbox).

Surrounding Structure: The ulnar branch of the medial branch of the superficial radial nerve is located on the ulnar (medial) side of the extensor pollicis longus tendon.

Additional Observation: The ulnar branch of the medial branch of the superficial radial nerve will supply the rest of the superficial branch of the radial nerve's distribution.

SECTION 4

Fig. 1 Deep Branch of Radial Nerve / Superficial Branch of Radial Nerve / Articular Cartilage of Anterior Elbow / Brachialis Muscle / Brachioradialis Muscle

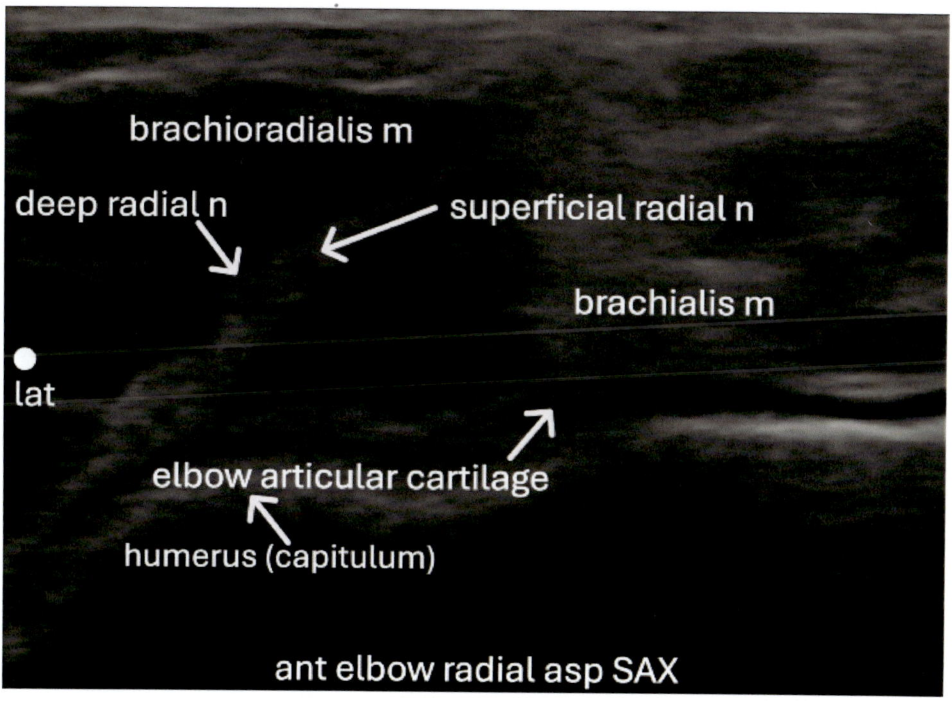

Probe Position: The probe is placed transversely (with its axis perpendicular to the arm) immediately proximal to the radial side of the elbow crease.

Anatomical Landmark: The anterior elbow articular cartilage at the capitulum of the humerus.

Surrounding Structures: The deep branch of the radial nerve, which will become the posterior interosseous nerve further distally, is located between the brachialis and brachioradialis muscles, and just deep to the superficial branch of the radial nerve.

Additional Observations: Scanning distally from this position reveals the deep branch of the radial nerve approaching the supinator muscle. The supinator muscle is located on the radius and becomes visible as the brachialis muscle moves distally towards its insertion on the ulna.

Fig. 2 Deep Branch of Radial Nerve / Deep and Superficial Layers of Supinator Muscle / Arcade of Frohse

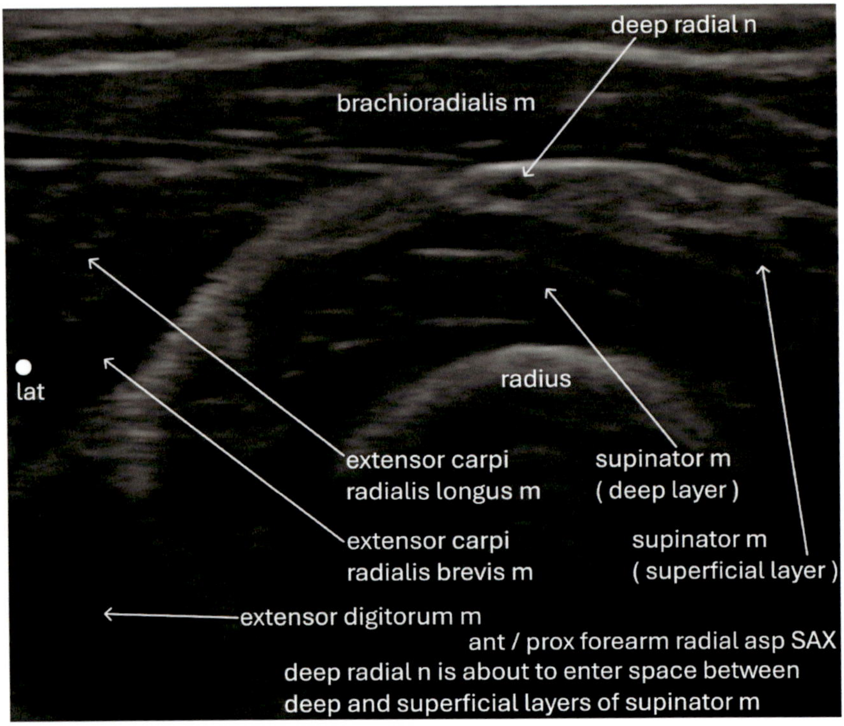

Probe Position: The probe is placed transversely on the radial side of the anterior, proximal forearm, distal to the location shown in Fig. 1.

Anatomical Landmark: The supinator muscle on the radius.

Surrounding Structures: At this point, the deep branch of the radial nerve is about to enter the space between the deep and superficial layers of the supinator muscle at the arcade of Frohse. This arcade is a tendinous or fibrous arch formed by the proximal edge of the superficial layer of the supinator muscle.

Additional Observations: The supinator muscle is surrounded by the brachioradialis, extensor carpi radialis longus, extensor carpi radialis brevis, and extensor digitorum muscles. At this level, the deep branch of the radial nerve is situated between the supinator and brachioradialis muscles.

Fig. 3 Posterior Interosseous Nerve / Deep and Superficial Layers of Supinator Muscle

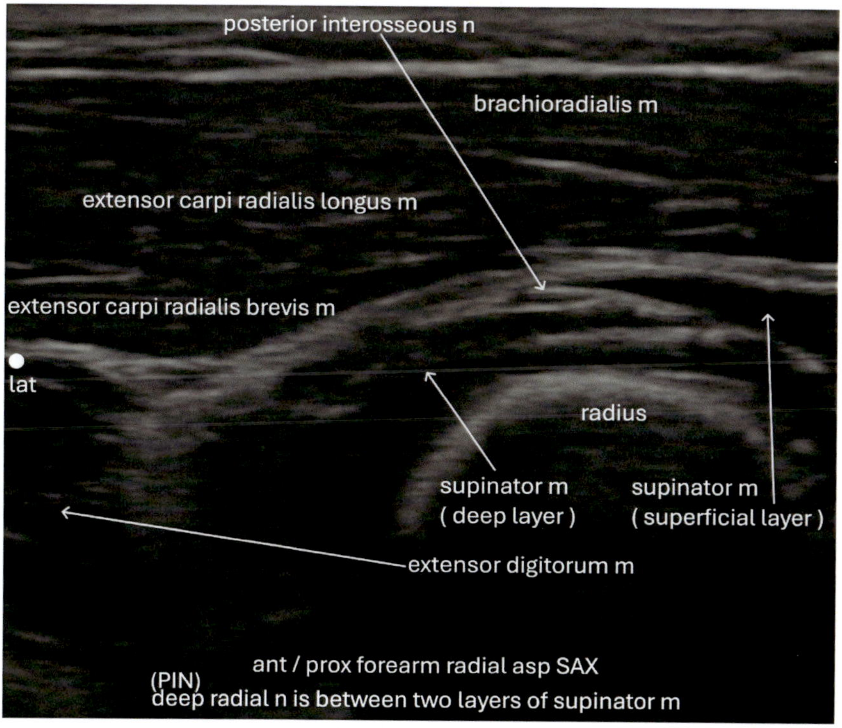

Probe Position: The probe is placed transversely on the radial side of the anterior, proximal forearm, just distal to the location shown in Fig. 2.

Anatomical Landmark: The supinator muscle on the radius.

Surrounding Structures: At this point, the deep branch of the radial nerve (posterior interosseous nerve) travels between the deep and superficial layers of the supinator muscle, just after passing through the arcade of Frohse.

Additional Observation: The supinator muscle is surrounded by the brachioradialis, extensor carpi radialis longus, extensor carpi radialis brevis, and extensor digitorum muscles.

Fig. 4 Posterior Interosseous Nerve / Deep and Superficial Layers of Supinator Muscle

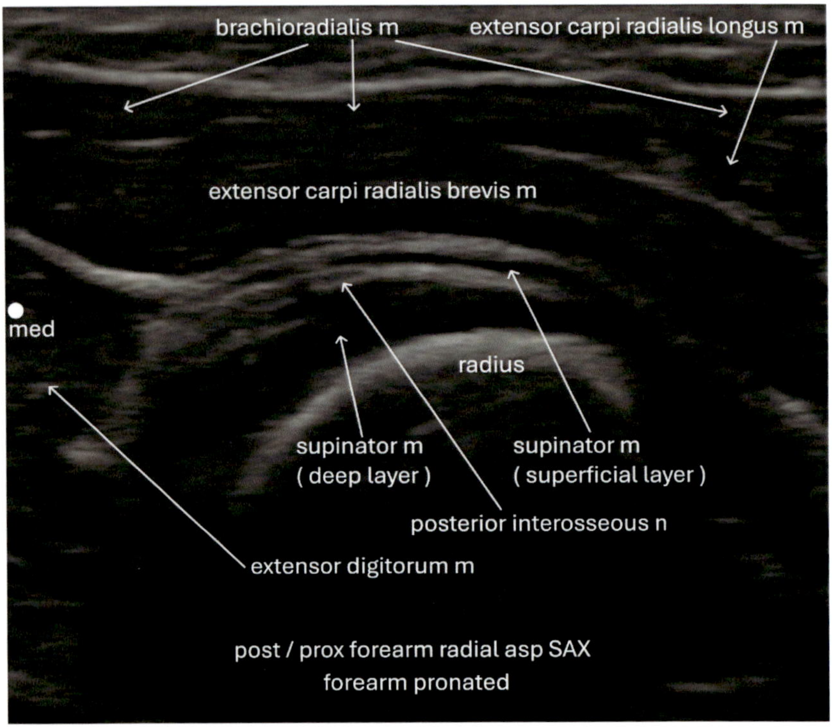

Probe Position: The probe is placed transversely on the radial side of the posterior, proximal forearm, just distal to the level shown in Fig. 3. As follows:
The probe is moved distally by crossing over the lateral (radial) edge of the forearm from the anterior to the posterior side while simultaneously pronating the forearm. The probe will then be positioned on the posterior aspect.

Anatomical Landmark: The supinator muscle on the radius.

Surrounding Structures: At this point, the posterior interosseous nerve is traveling between the deep and superficial layers of the supinator muscle.

Additional Observation: The supinator muscle is surrounded by the extensor carpi radialis brevis and extensor digitorum muscles.

Fig. 5 Posterior Interosseous Nerve / Supinator Muscle / Extensor Digitorum Muscle

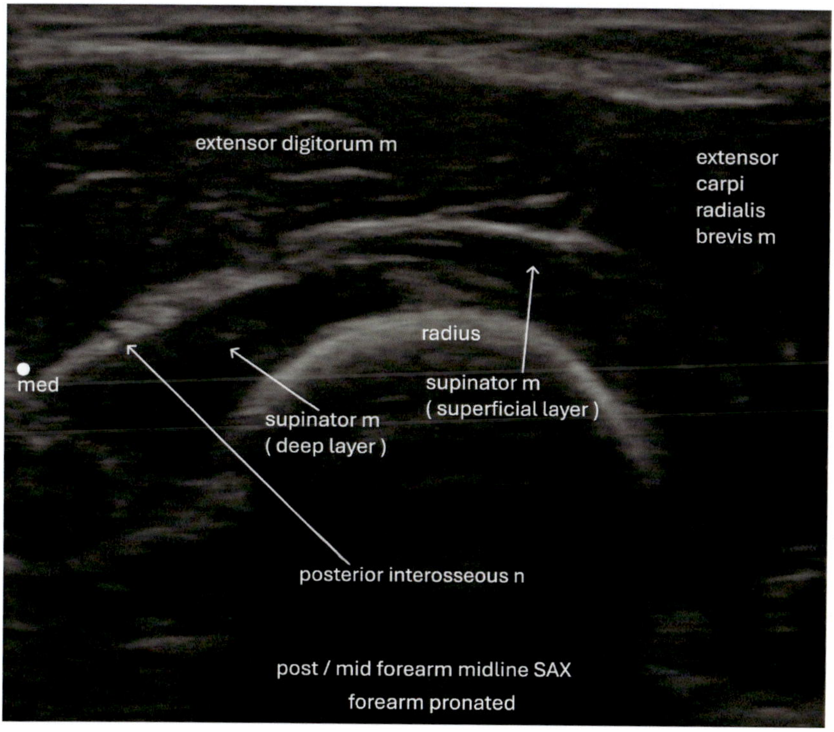

Probe Position: The probe is placed transversely on the midline of the posterior, mid-forearm, just distal to the level shown in Fig. 4. The forearm is pronated.

Anatomical Landmark: The supinator muscle on the radius.

Surrounding Structures: The posterior interosseous nerve, immediately after exiting the supinator muscle, divides into multiple branches that supply the muscles of the posterior forearm.

Additional Observation: The supinator muscle is surrounded by the extensor carpi radialis brevis and extensor digitorum muscles.

Fig. 6 Posterior Interosseous Nerve / Supinator Muscle / Abductor Pollicis Longus Muscle / Extensor Digitorum Muscle / Extensor Digiti Minimi Muscle / Extensor Carpi Ulnaris Muscle

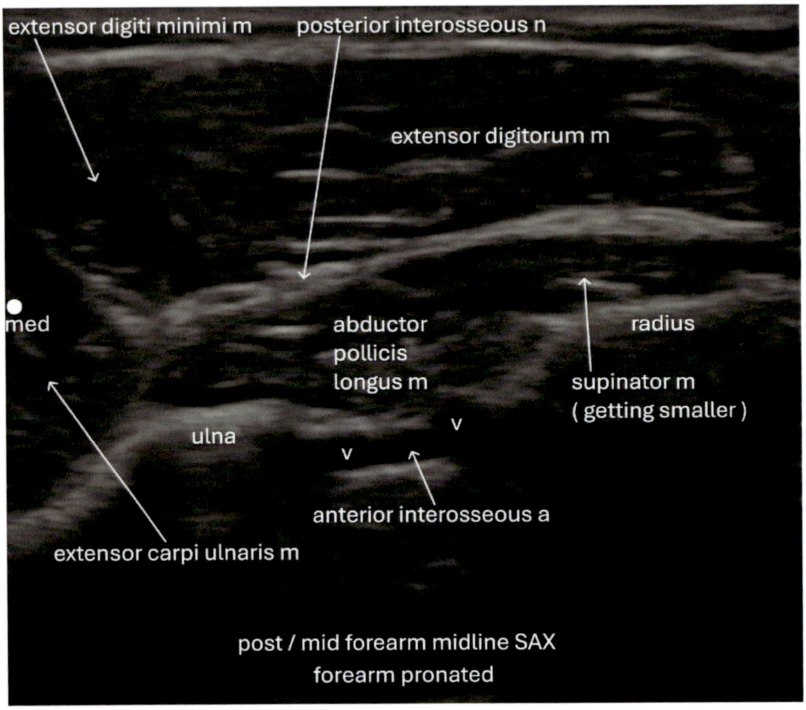

Probe Position: The probe is placed transversely on the midline of the posterior, mid-forearm, just distal to the level shown in Fig. 5. The forearm is pronated.

Anatomical Landmarks: The abductor pollicis longus muscle and the anterior interosseous artery, which is located just deep to the interosseous membrane between the ulna and radius bones.

Surrounding Structure: The branches of the posterior interosseous nerve are located on the superficial surface of the abductor pollicis longus muscle.

Additional Observations: The supinator muscle is decreasing in size, while the abductor pollicis longus muscle appears medial (ulnar) to it. Between the extensor digitorum and extensor carpi ulnaris muscles is the extensor digiti minimi muscle, which becomes visible just after the anconeus muscle goes out of view. The anconeus muscle on the ulnar side is not shown in this image. Additionally, the brachioradialis, extensor carpi radialis longus, and extensor carpi radialis brevis muscles are outside the field of view.

Fig. 7 Posterior Interosseous Nerve / Abductor Pollicis Longus Muscle / Extensor Pollicis Brevis Muscle / Extensor Pollicis Longus Muscle

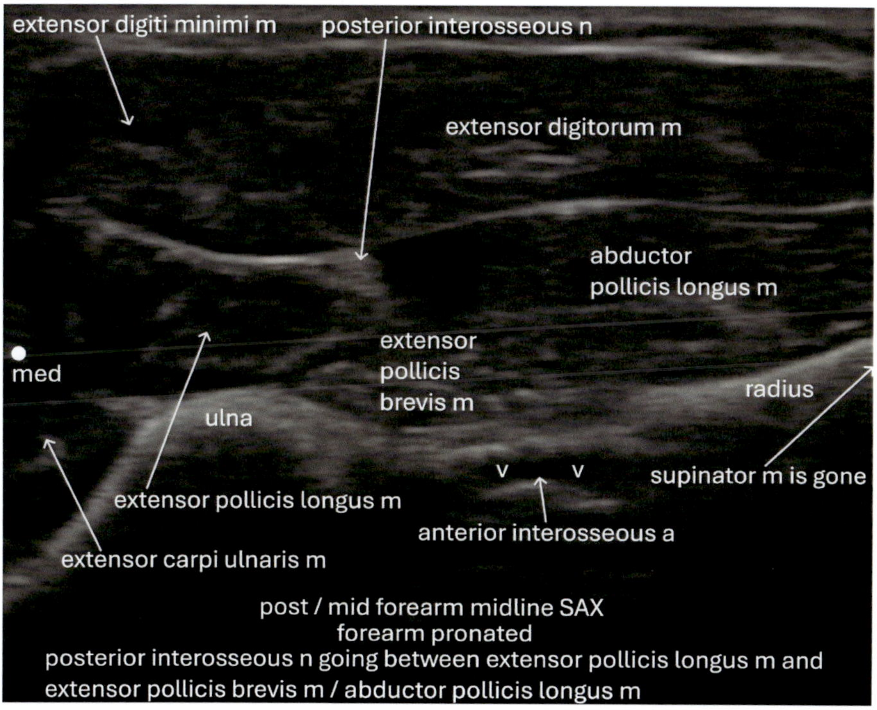

Probe Position: The probe is placed transversely on the midline of the posterior, mid-forearm, just distal to the level shown in Fig. 6. The forearm is pronated.

Anatomical Landmark: The extensor pollicis longus muscle is located on the ulna.

Surrounding Structures: The deep branches of the posterior interosseous nerve run in the superficial space between the abductor pollicis longus and extensor pollicis longus muscles.

Additional Observations: The abductor pollicis longus muscle is on the radius, and the supinator muscle is no longer visible at this point. The extensor pollicis brevis muscle can be seen just superficial to the interosseous membrane between the ulna and radius, while the extensor pollicis longus muscle begins to appear on the ulna.

Fig. 8 Posterior Interosseous Nerve / Extensor Pollicis Brevis Muscle / Extensor Pollicis Longus Muscle / Extensor Indicis Muscle

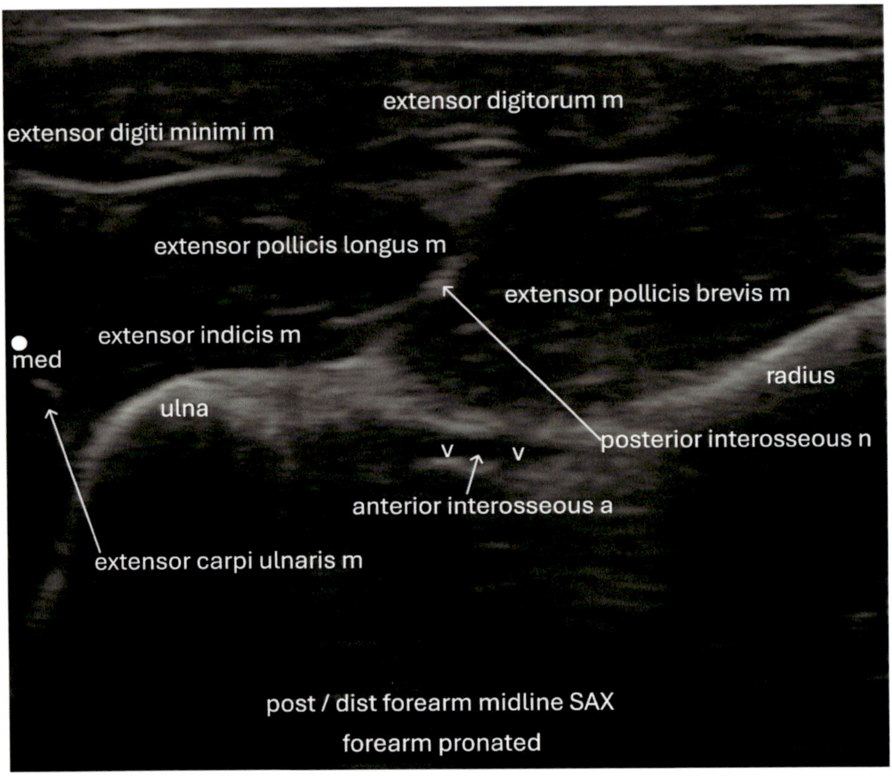

Probe Position: The probe is placed transversely on the midline of the posterior, distal forearm, just distal to the level shown in Fig. 7. The forearm is pronated.

Anatomical Landmark: The extensor indicis muscle is located on the ulna.

Surrounding Structures: The deep branches of the posterior interosseous nerve run between the extensor pollicis brevis and extensor pollicis longus muscles.

Additional Observations: The abductor pollicis longus muscle goes out of view, and the extensor pollicis brevis muscle is on the radius. The extensor indicis muscle begins to appear on the ulna.

Fig. 9 Posterior Interosseous Nerve / Extensor Pollicis Brevis Muscle / Extensor Pollicis Longus Muscle / Extensor Indicis Muscle / Interosseous Membrane

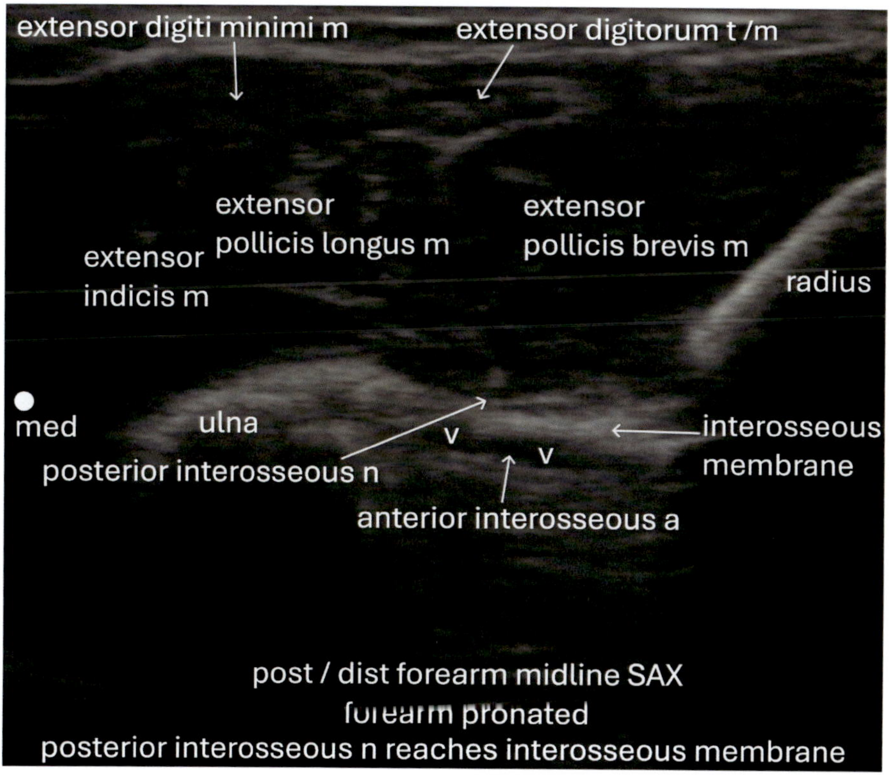

Probe Position: The probe is placed transversely on the midline of the posterior, distal forearm, just distal to the level shown in Fig. 8. The forearm is pronated.

Anatomical Landmark: The interosseous membrane between the ulna and radius.

Surrounding Structure: The posterior interosseous nerve reaches the interosseous membrane. It then runs along the membrane to the dorsal aspect of the wrist, where its terminal branch innervates the wrist joint capsule and ligaments with sensory fibers (proprioception, which is the sense of joint position and movement). It does not innervate the skin.

Additional Observation: The musculotendinous junction of the extensor digitorum is visible.

Fig. 10 Extensor Pollicis Brevis Muscle / Extensor Pollicis Longus Muscle / Extensor Indicis Muscle / Interosseous Membrane

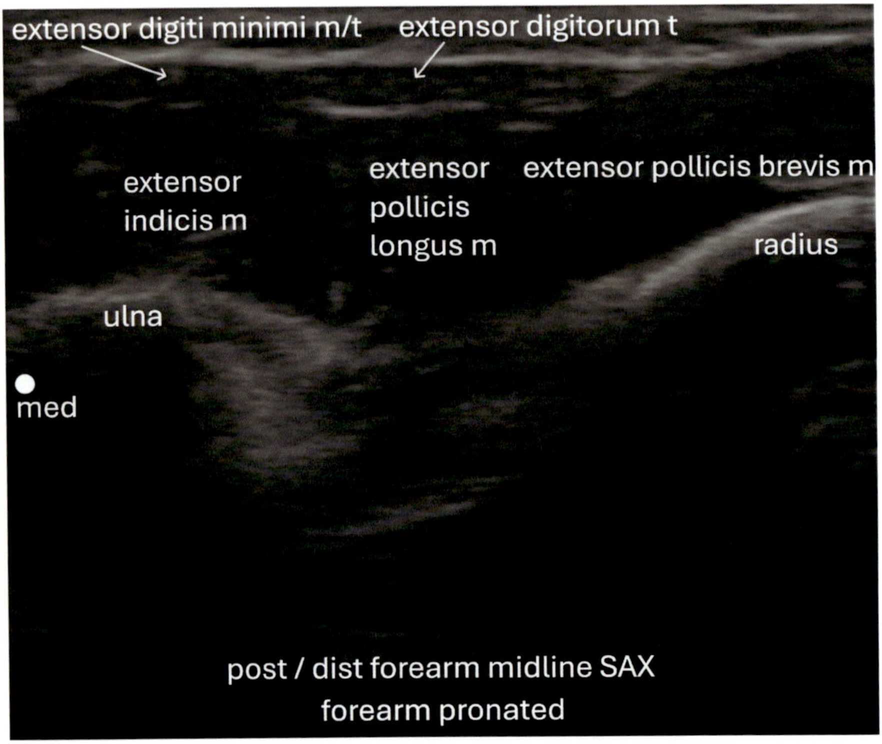

Probe Position: The probe is placed transversely on the midline of the posterior, distal forearm, just distal to the level shown in Fig. 9. The forearm is pronated.

Anatomical Landmark: The interosseous membrane between the ulna and radius.

Surrounding Structure: Tracing the posterior interosseous nerve from this level is difficult, but it can be done. (Not shown here)

Additional Observations: The extensor pollicis brevis muscle is on the radius. The extensor indicis muscle is on the ulna, and the extensor pollicis longus muscle is visible superficial to the interosseous membrane between the ulna and radius. The musculotendinous junction of the extensor digiti minimi is also visible.

Fig. 11 Extensor Pollicis Brevis Muscle / Musculotendinous Junction of Extensor Pollicis Longus / Extensor Indicis Muscle

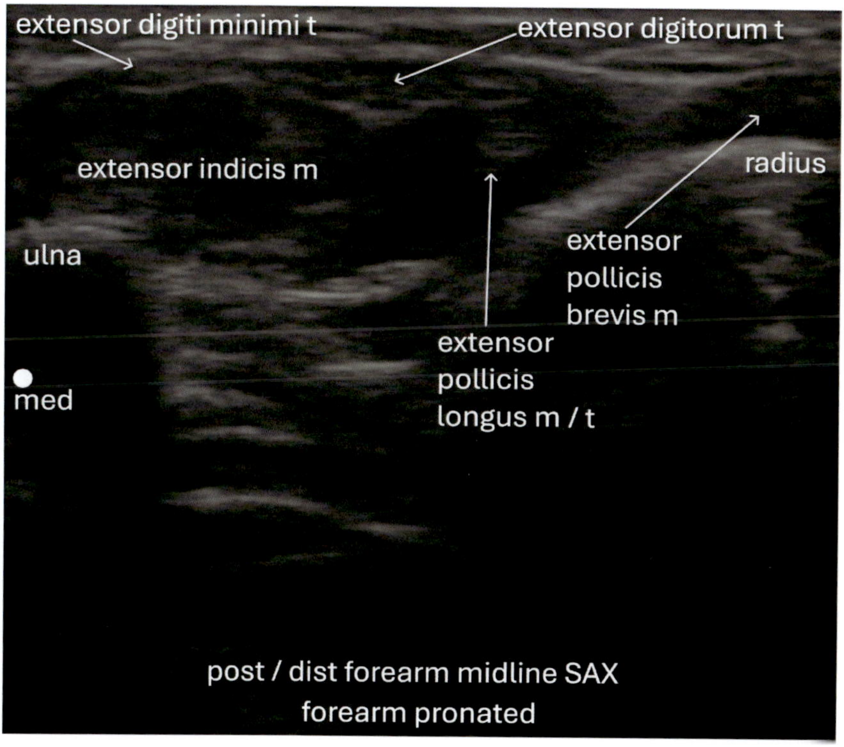

Probe Position: The probe is placed transversely on the midline of the posterior, distal forearm, just distal to the level shown in Fig. 10. The forearm is pronated.

Anatomical Landmarks: The ulna and radius.

Visualized Structures: The extensor pollicis brevis muscle passes radially on the radius. The musculotendinous junction of the extensor pollicis longus comes to lie on the radius. The extensor indicis is located on the ulnar side.

Other Structures: The extensor digitorum and extensor digiti minimi tendons are visible superficially.

Fig. 12 Extensor Pollicis Brevis Muscle / Extensor Pollicis Longus Tendon / Musculotendinous Junction of Extensor Indicis

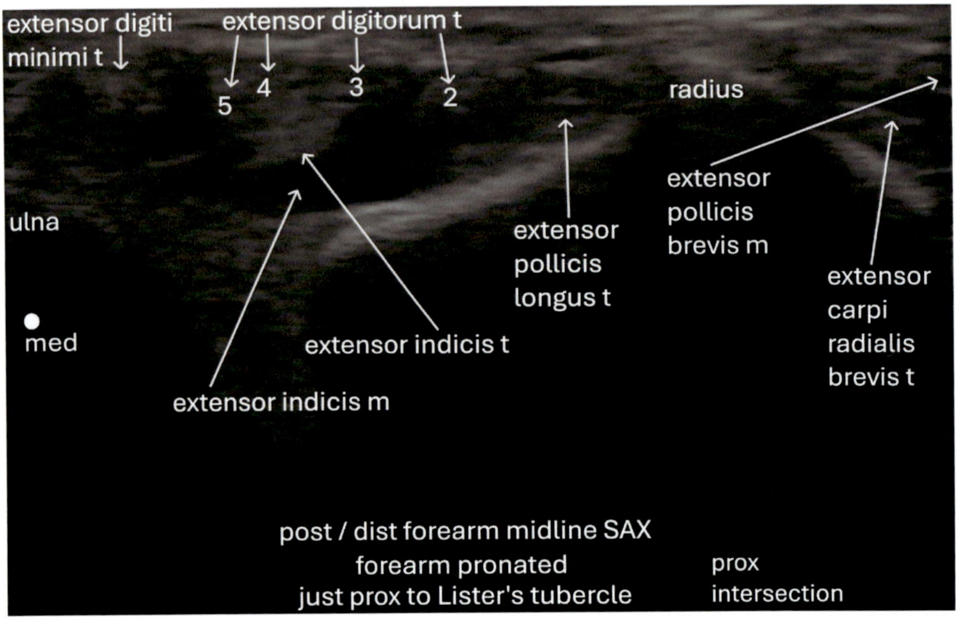

Probe Position: The probe is placed transversely on the midline of the posterior, distal forearm, just distal to the level shown in Fig. 11. The forearm is pronated.

Anatomical Landmark: The radius just proximal to Lister's tubercle.

Visualized Structures: The musculotendinous junction of the extensor indicis is located just deep to the extensor digitorum tendons, which are now visible as individual tendons of the digits. The extensor digiti minimi tendon is visible ulnar to the extensor digitorum tendon.

Additional Observations: The extensor pollicis brevis muscle passes over the extensor carpi radialis brevis tendon, forming the proximal intersection. The extensor pollicis longus tendon lies on the radius.

Fig. 13 Lister's Tubercle of Radius / Extensor Pollicis Longus Tendon / Musculotendinous Junction of Extensor Indicis

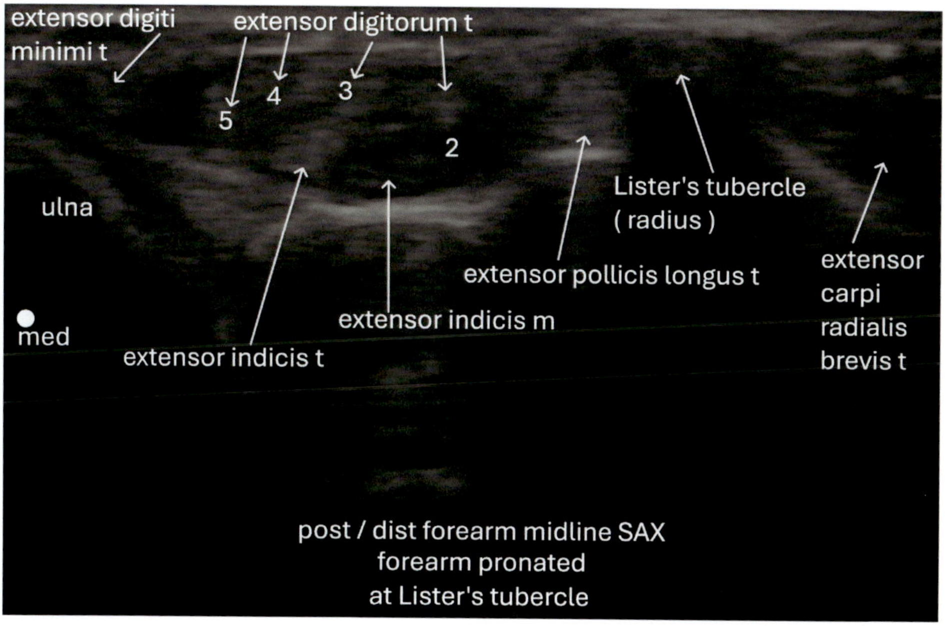

Probe Position: The probe is placed transversely on the midline of the posterior, distal forearm, just distal to the level shown in Fig. 12. The forearm is pronated.

Anatomical Landmark: Lister's tubercle of the radius.

Visualized Structures: The musculotendinous junction of the extensor indicis is located just deep to the extensor digitorum tendons. The extensor digiti minimi tendon is visible ulnar to the extensor digitorum tendon.

Additional Observations: The extensor pollicis brevis muscle went out of view. The extensor pollicis longus tendon lies just ulnar (medial) to Lister's tubercle of the radius.

Fig. 14 Proximal Carpal Bones / Distal Intersection / Extensor Pollicis Longus Tendon / Musculotendinous Junction of Extensor Indicis

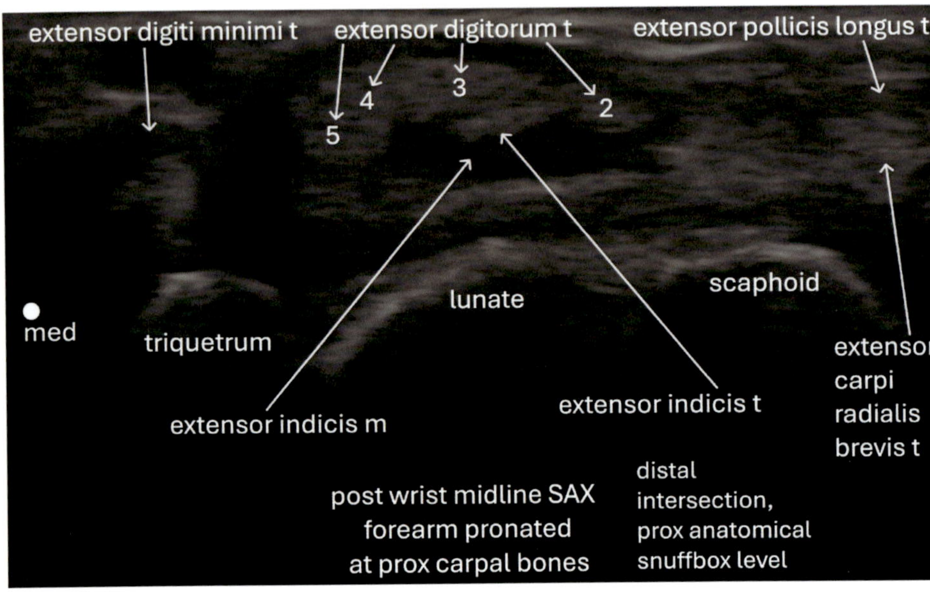

Probe Position: The probe is placed transversely on the midline of the posterior wrist, just distal to the level shown in Fig. 13. The forearm is pronated.

Anatomical Landmarks: At the level of the proximal part of the anatomical snuffbox, proximal carpal bones are visible by placing ultrasound probe on the dorsal wrist.

Visualized Structures: The musculotendinous junction of the extensor indicis is located just deep to the extensor digitorum tendons. The extensor digiti minimi tendon is visible ulnar to the extensor digitorum tendon.

Additional Observation: The extensor pollicis longus tendon courses radially and is situated over the extensor carpi radialis brevis tendon, forming the distal intersection.

Fig. 15 Distal Carpal Bones / Extensor Indicis Tendon

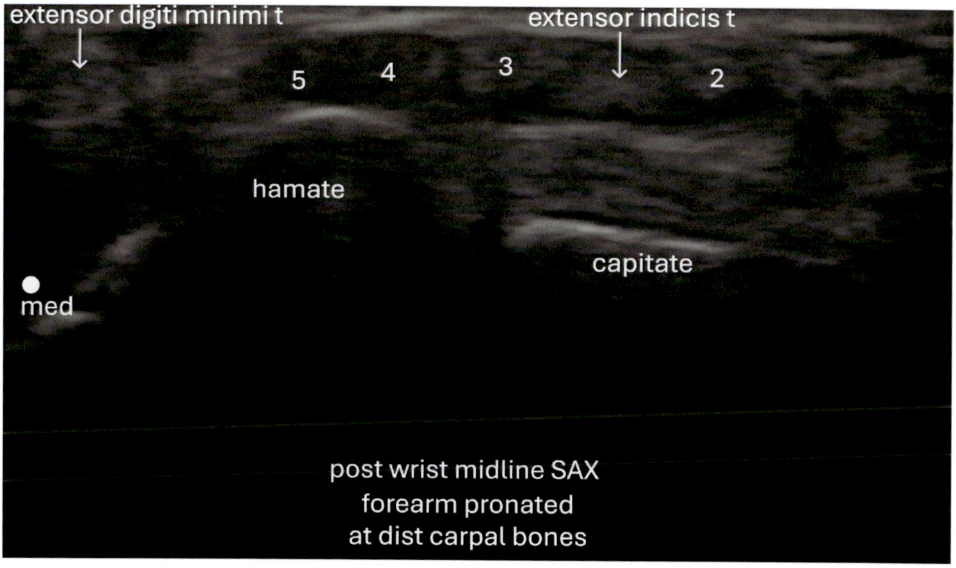

Probe Position: The probe is placed transversely on the midline of the posterior wrist, just distal to the level shown in Fig. 14. The forearm is pronated.

Anatomical Landmarks: The capitate and hamate.

Visualized Structures: The extensor indicis tendon is located between the extensor digitorum tendons for the 2nd and 3rd digits. The extensor digiti minimi tendon is visible ulnar to the extensor digitorum tendon.

Additional Observation: The extensor pollicis longus tendon is not shown in this view.

Fig. 16 Extensor Digitorum Muscle / Extensor Carpi Ulnaris Muscle / Anconeus Muscle

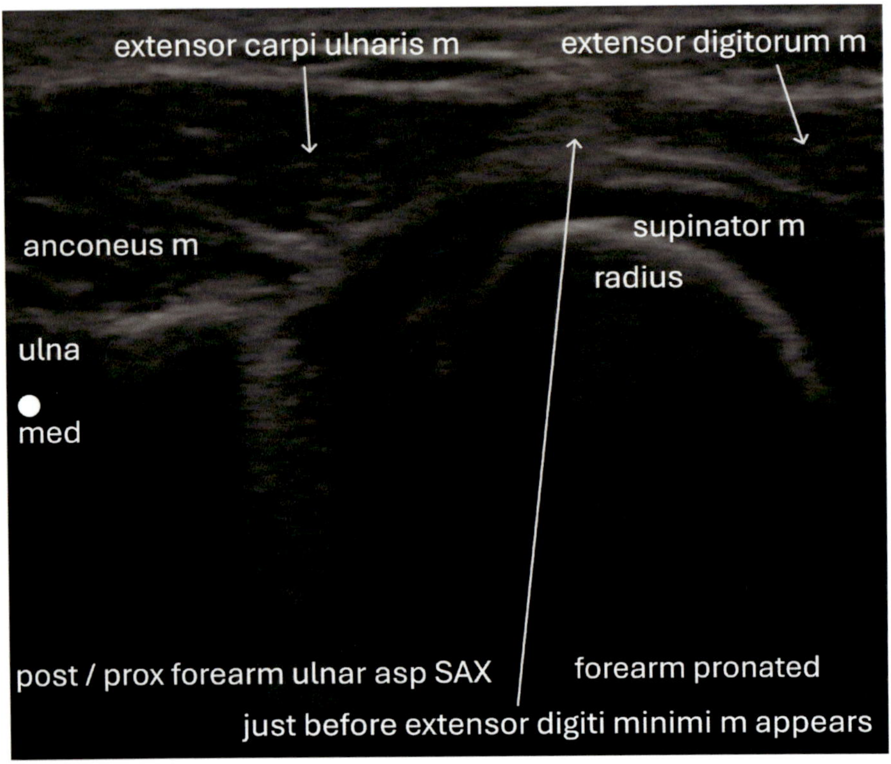

Probe Position: The probe is placed transversely, slightly on the ulnar side of the posterior, proximal forearm. The forearm is pronated.

Anatomical Landmark: The anconeus muscle is located on the ulna.

Visualized Structures: From the radial to the ulnar side, the extensor digitorum, extensor carpi ulnaris, and anconeus muscles are visible.

Additional Observation: The extensor digiti minimi muscle is not yet visible between the extensor digitorum and extensor carpi ulnaris muscles.

Fig. 17 Extensor Digitorum Muscle / Extensor Digiti Minimi Muscle / Extensor Carpi Ulnaris Muscle

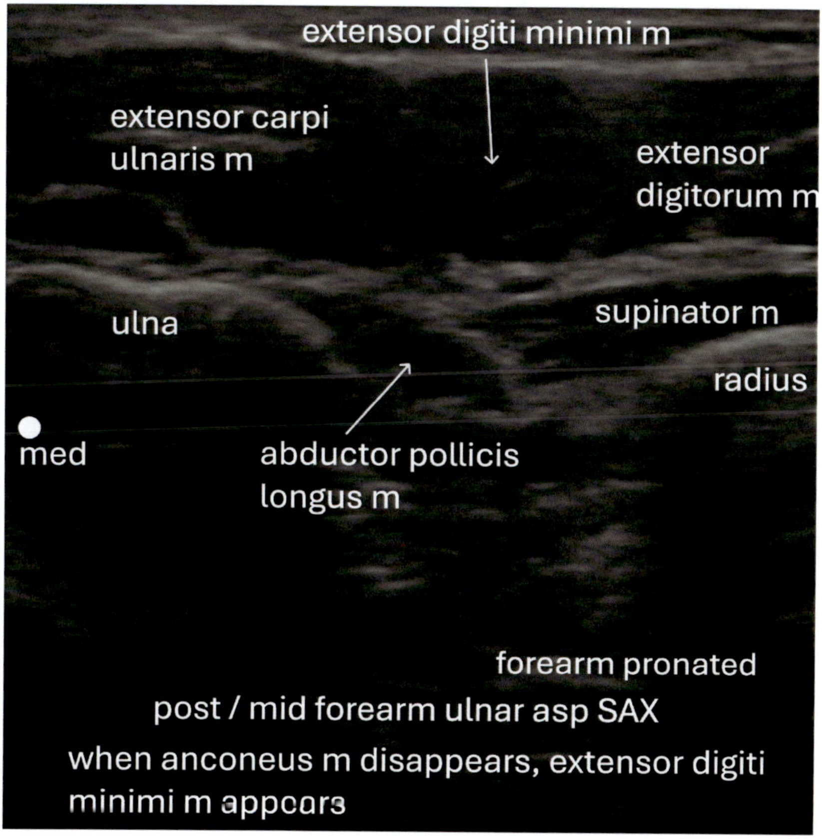

Probe Position: The probe is placed transversely on the ulnar side of the posterior, mid-forearm, just distal to the level shown in Fig. 16. The forearm is pronated.

Anatomical Landmark: The anconeus muscle is no longer visible.

Visualized Structures: From the radial to the ulnar side, the extensor digitorum, extensor digiti minimi, and extensor carpi ulnaris muscles are visible.

Additional Observation: As soon as the anconeus muscle is no longer visible, the extensor digiti minimi muscle becomes visible between the extensor digitorum and extensor carpi ulnaris muscles.

SECTION 5

Fig. 1 Ulnar Nerve / Medial Epicondyle / Olecranon / Cubital Tunnel

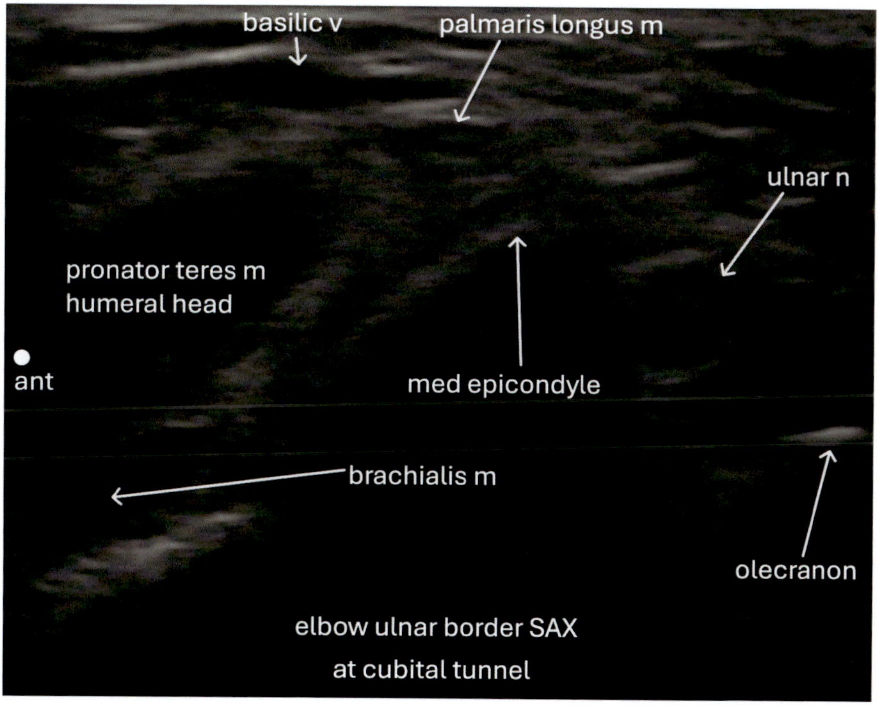

Probe Position: The probe is placed transversely on the ulnar border of the elbow, between the anterior and posterior aspects.

Anatomical Landmarks: The medial epicondyle and the olecranon.

Surrounding Structures: The ulnar nerve is located in the cubital tunnel, between the medial epicondyle and the olecranon.

Additional Observations: The palmaris longus and the humeral head of the pronator teres muscles can be visible. The basilic vein is also located superficially.

Fig. 2 Ulnar Nerve / Humeral and Ulnar Heads of Flexor Carpi Ulnaris Muscle / Flexor Digitorum Superficialis and Profundus Muscles / Palmaris Longus Muscle / Flexor Carpi Radialis Muscle / Humeral Head of Pronator Teres Muscle

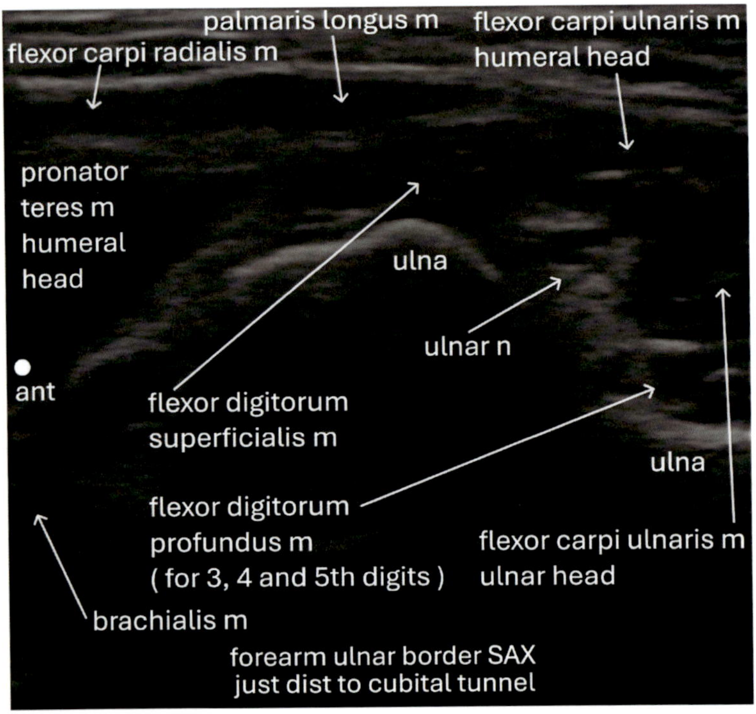

Probe Position: The probe is placed transversely on the ulnar border of the proximal forearm, just distal to the location shown in Fig. 1 (just distal to the cubital tunnel).

Anatomical Landmarks: The humeral and ulnar heads of the flexor carpi ulnaris muscle.

Surrounding Structures: The ulnar nerve is located between the two heads of the flexor carpi ulnaris muscle, close to the ulna.

Additional Observations: In addition to the palmaris longus and the humeral head of the pronator teres muscles, the flexor carpi radialis, the two heads of the flexor carpi ulnaris, and the humeroulnar head of the flexor digitorum superficialis muscles also start to become visible. Additionally, the flexor digitorum profundus muscle for the 3rd, 4th, and 5th digits starts to appear on the ulna, deep to the flexor carpi ulnaris muscle.

Fig. 3 Ulnar Nerve / Flexor Carpi Ulnaris Muscle / Flexor Digitorum Superficialis and Profundus Muscles / Palmaris Longus Muscle

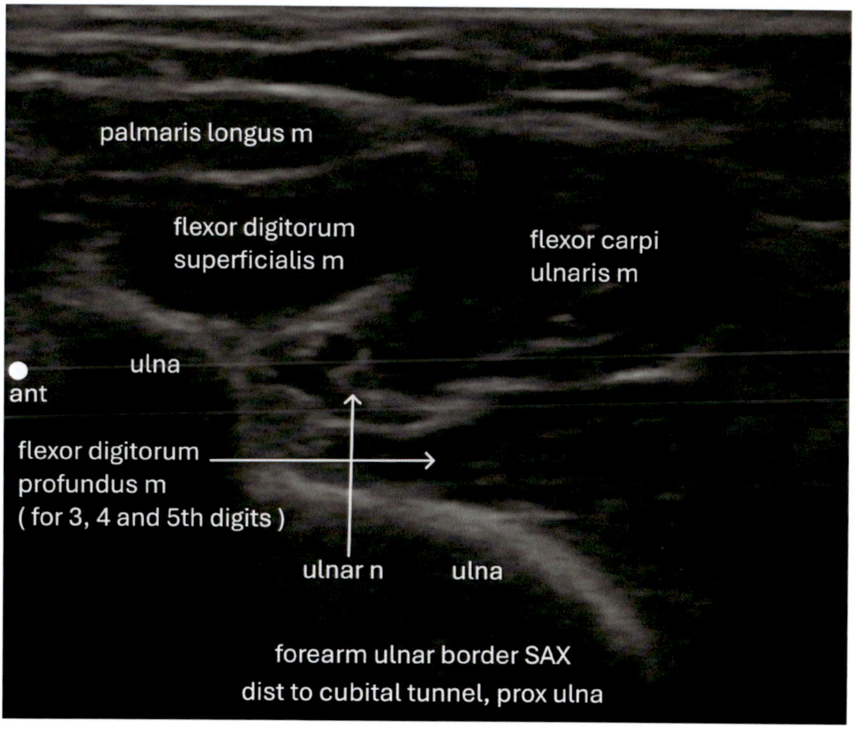

Probe Position: The probe is placed transversely on the ulnar border of the proximal forearm, just distal to the location shown in Fig. 2 (distal to the cubital tunnel).

Anatomical Landmark: The two heads of the flexor carpi ulnaris (the humeral head and the ulnar head) merge to form a single muscle belly.

Surrounding Structures: The ulnar nerve is located between the flexor carpi ulnaris muscle and the ulna, also situated between the flexor digitorum superficialis and profundus muscles.

Additional Observation: The palmaris longus muscle is visible superficially.

Fig. 4 Ulnar Nerve / Flexor Carpi Ulnaris Muscle / Flexor Digitorum Superficialis and Profundus Muscles / Ulnar Head of Pronator Teres Muscle

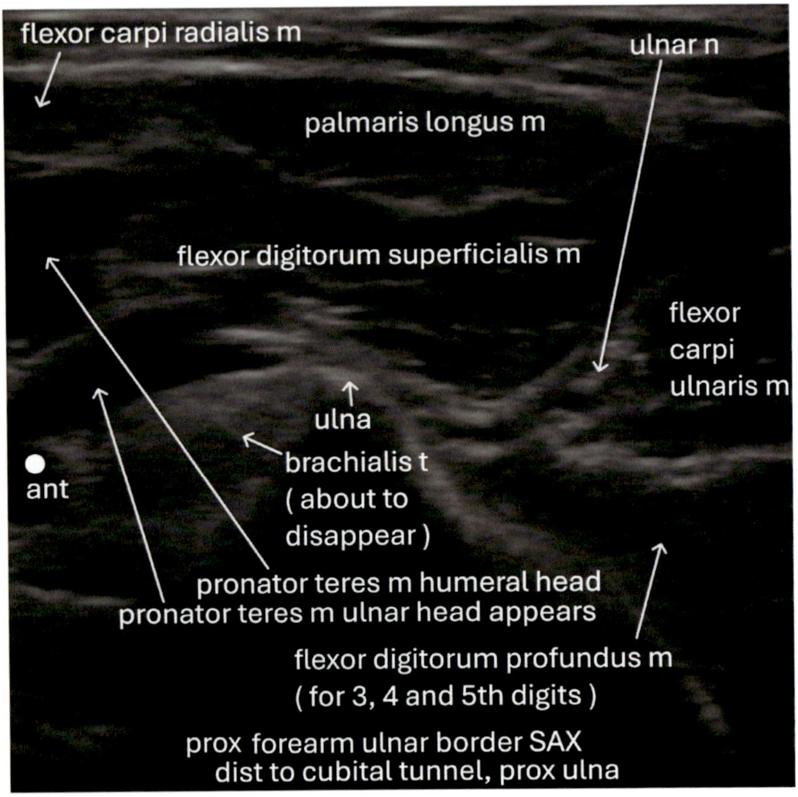

Probe Position: The probe is placed transversely on the ulnar border of the proximal forearm, just distal to the location shown in Fig. 3 (distal to the cubital tunnel).

Anatomical Landmark: The flexor carpi ulnaris muscle.

Surrounding Structures: The ulnar nerve is enveloped by the flexor carpi ulnaris, the flexor digitorum superficialis, and the flexor digitorum profundus muscles.

Additional Observations: In this view, the flexor carpi radialis and the humeral head of the pronator teres muscles are shown. Deep to that, the ulnar head of the pronator teres muscle starts to appear as the brachialis muscle moves out of view to its insertion.

Fig. 5 Ulnar Nerve / Flexor Carpi Ulnaris Muscle / Flexor Digitorum Superficialis and Profundus Muscles / Median Nerve / Ulnar Artery

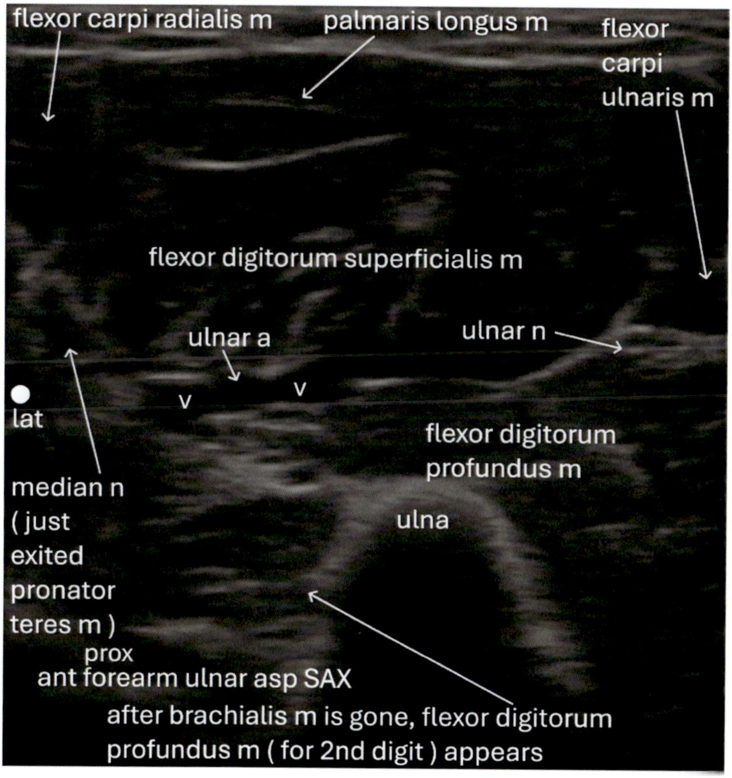

Probe Position: The probe is placed transversely on the ulnar side of the proximal anterior forearm, just distal to the location shown in Fig. 4.

Anatomical Landmark: The flexor carpi ulnaris muscle.

Surrounding Structures: The ulnar nerve is enveloped by the flexor carpi ulnaris, the flexor digitorum superficialis, and the flexor digitorum profundus muscles.

Additional Observations: This view shows the median nerve as it emerges from the pronator teres muscle, which lies outside the image field on the left. Once the brachialis muscle goes out of view, the flexor digitorum profundus muscle for the second digit becomes visible on the lateral side of the ulna. Here, the entire flexor digitorum profundus muscle appears to be covering the ulna, and the ulnar artery is still close to the median nerve.

Fig. 6 Flexor Digitorum Superficialis and Profundus Muscles / Median Nerve / Ulnar Artery

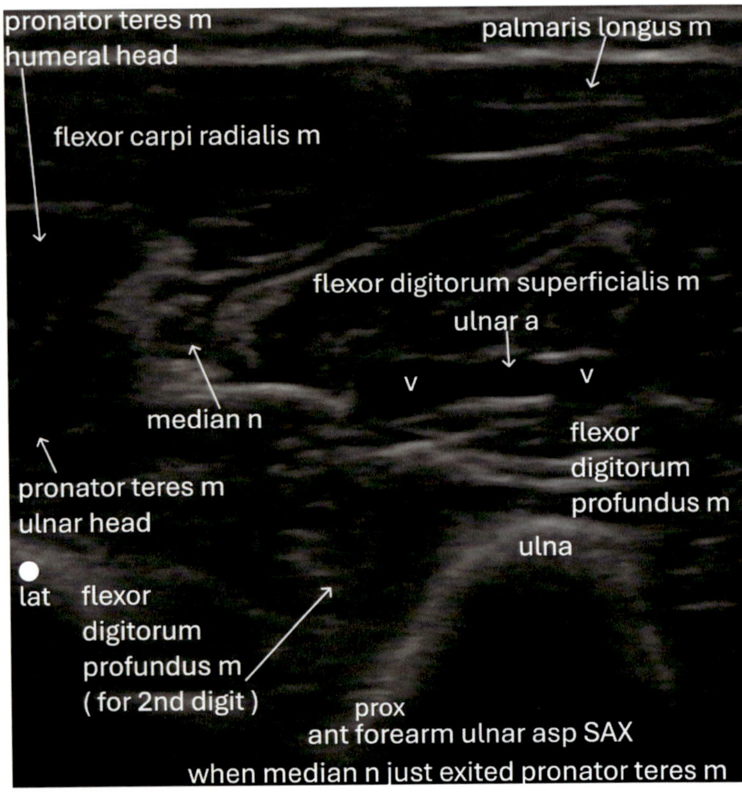

Probe Position: The probe is placed transversely on the ulnar side of the proximal anterior forearm, just distal to the location shown in Fig. 5.

Anatomical Landmark: The ulnar artery.

Visualized Structures: The ulnar nerve lies outside the image field on the right. The ulnar artery is positioned slightly away from the median nerve, located between the flexor digitorum superficialis and profundus muscles.

Additional Observations: The pronator teres muscle is visible on the left. The palmaris longus and flexor carpi radialis muscles are seen superficially. The flexor digitorum profundus muscle is located on the ulna.

Fig. 7 Ulnar Nerve / Flexor Carpi Ulnaris Muscle / Flexor Digitorum Superficialis and Profundus Muscles

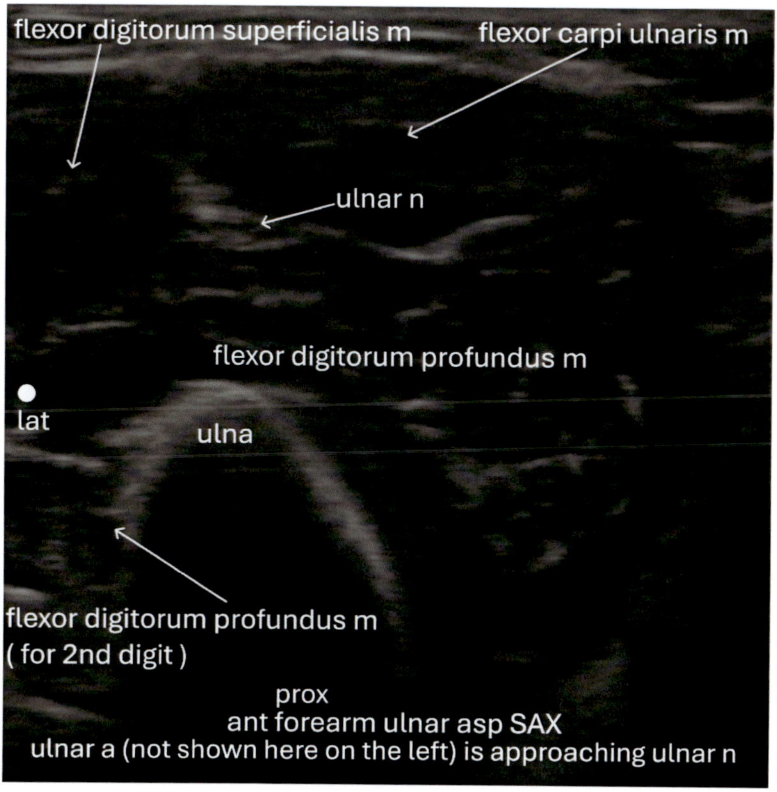

Probe Position: The probe is placed transversely on the ulnar side of the proximal anterior forearm, at the same level as the location shown in Fig. 6, but more to the ulnar aspect.

Anatomical Landmark: The flexor carpi ulnaris muscle.

Surrounding Structures: The ulnar artery lies outside the image field on the left. The ulnar nerve is enveloped by the flexor carpi ulnaris, the flexor digitorum superficialis, and the flexor digitorum profundus muscles.

Additional Observation: The medial aspect of the flexor carpi ulnaris and flexor digitorum profundus muscles can be seen better in this image.

Fig. 8 Ulnar Nerve / Flexor Carpi Ulnaris Muscle / Flexor Digitorum Superficialis and Profundus Muscles / Ulnar Artery

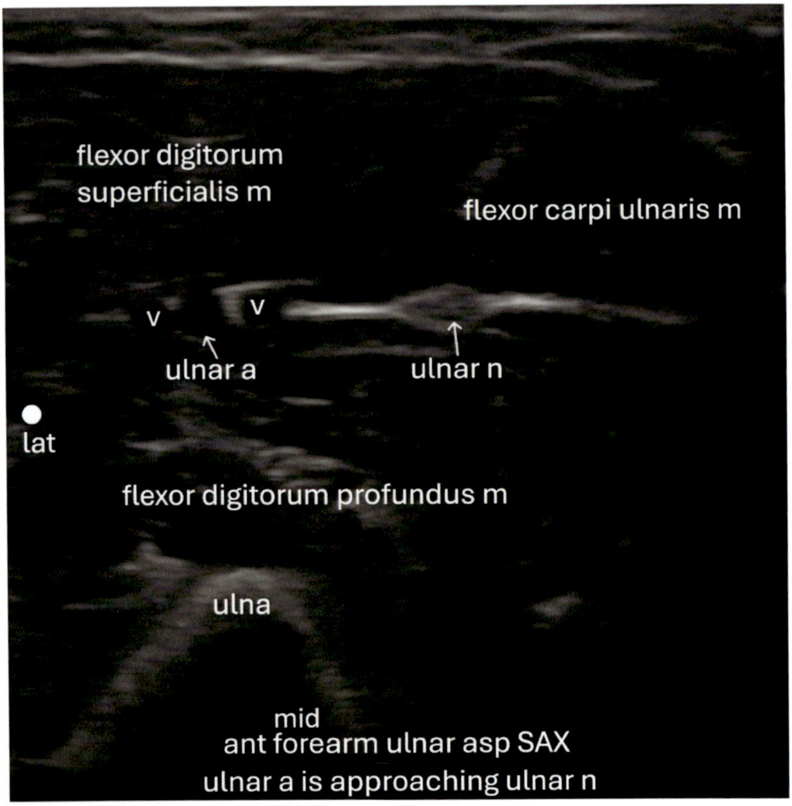

Probe Position: The probe is placed transversely on the ulnar side of the anterior mid-forearm, just distal to the location shown in Fig. 7.

Anatomical Landmark: The ulnar artery.

Surrounding Structures: The ulnar artery is approaching the ulnar nerve, which is enveloped by the flexor carpi ulnaris, the flexor digitorum superficialis, and the flexor digitorum profundus muscles.

Additional Observation: The ulnar artery is positioned between the flexor digitorum superficialis and profundus muscles.

Fig. 9 Ulnar Nerve / Flexor Carpi Ulnaris Muscle / Flexor Digitorum Superficialis and Profundus Muscles / Ulnar Artery / Ulnar Vein

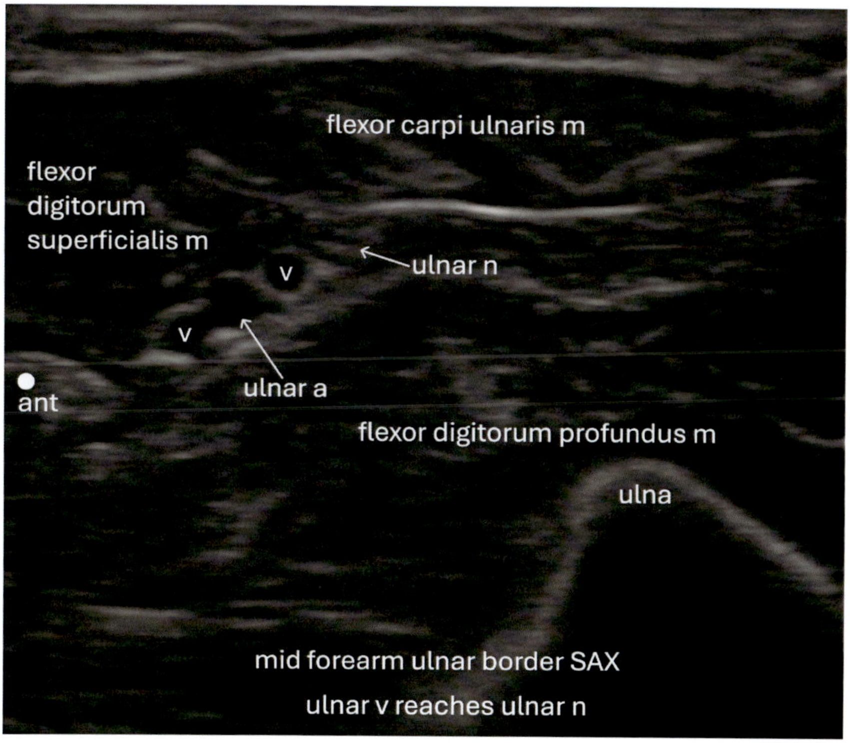

Probe Position: The probe is placed transversely on the ulnar border of the mid-forearm, between the anterior and posterior aspects, just distal to the location shown in Fig. 8.

Anatomical Landmark: The ulnar vein.

Surrounding Structures: The ulnar vein is just adjacent to the ulnar nerve, which is enveloped by the flexor carpi ulnaris, the flexor digitorum superficialis, and the flexor digitorum profundus muscles.

Additional Observation: From this level inferiorly, the ulnar artery and the ulnar nerve travel together side by side.

Fig. 10 Ulnar Nerve / Flexor Carpi Ulnaris Muscle / Flexor Digitorum Superficialis and Profundus Muscles / Ulnar Artery / Ulnar Vein

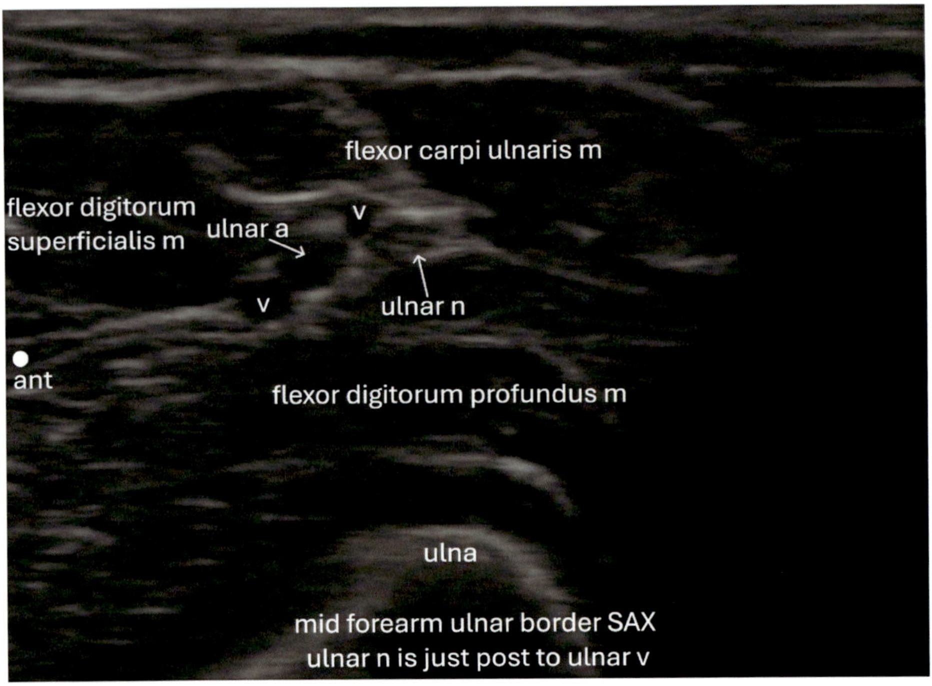

Probe Position: The probe is placed transversely on the ulnar border of the mid-forearm, just distal to the location shown in Fig. 9.

Anatomical Landmark: The ulnar vein.

Surrounding Structure: The ulnar nerve is situated just medial to the ulnar vein.

Additional Observations: The flexor carpi ulnaris, the flexor digitorum superficialis, and the flexor digitorum profundus muscles are visible.

Fig. 11 Palmar Cutaneous Branch of Ulnar Nerve / Ulnar Nerve / Flexor Carpi Ulnaris Muscle / Flexor Digitorum Superficialis and Profundus Muscles / Ulnar Artery / Ulnar Vein

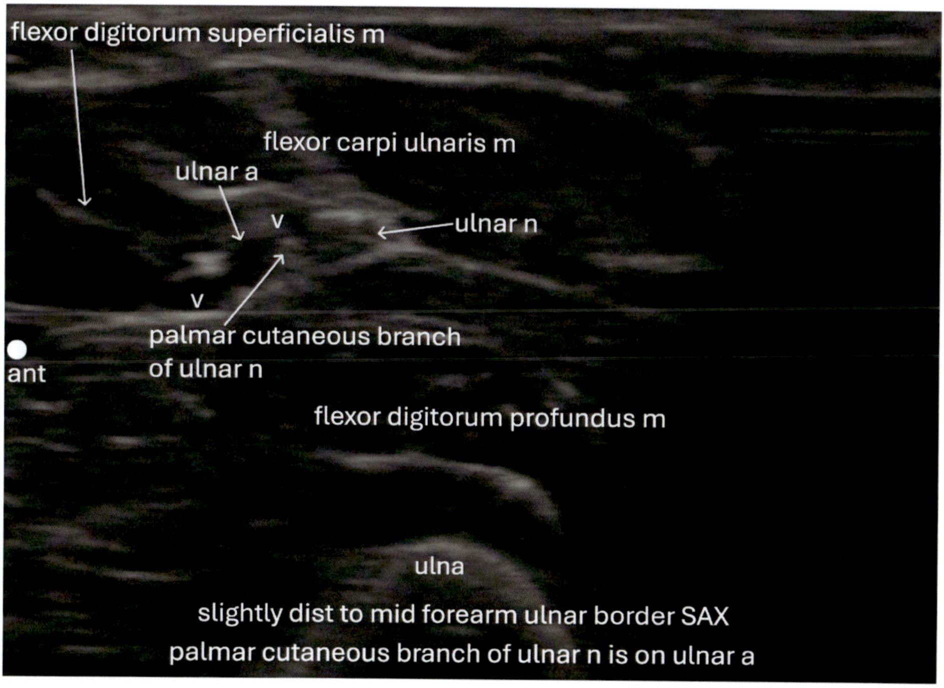

Probe Position: The probe is placed transversely on the ulnar border of the mid-forearm, just distal to the location shown in Fig. 10.

Anatomical Landmark: The ulnar artery.

Surrounding Structures: The ulnar nerve is situated just medial to the ulnar artery. The origin of the palmar cutaneous branch of the ulnar nerve may be visible between the ulnar nerve and the ulnar artery.

Additional Observations: The flexor carpi ulnaris, the flexor digitorum superficialis, and the flexor digitorum profundus muscles are visible.

Fig. 12 Palmar Cutaneous Branch of Ulnar Nerve / Ulnar Nerve / Flexor Carpi Ulnaris Muscle / Flexor Digitorum Superficialis and Profundus Muscles / Ulnar Artery / Ulnar Vein

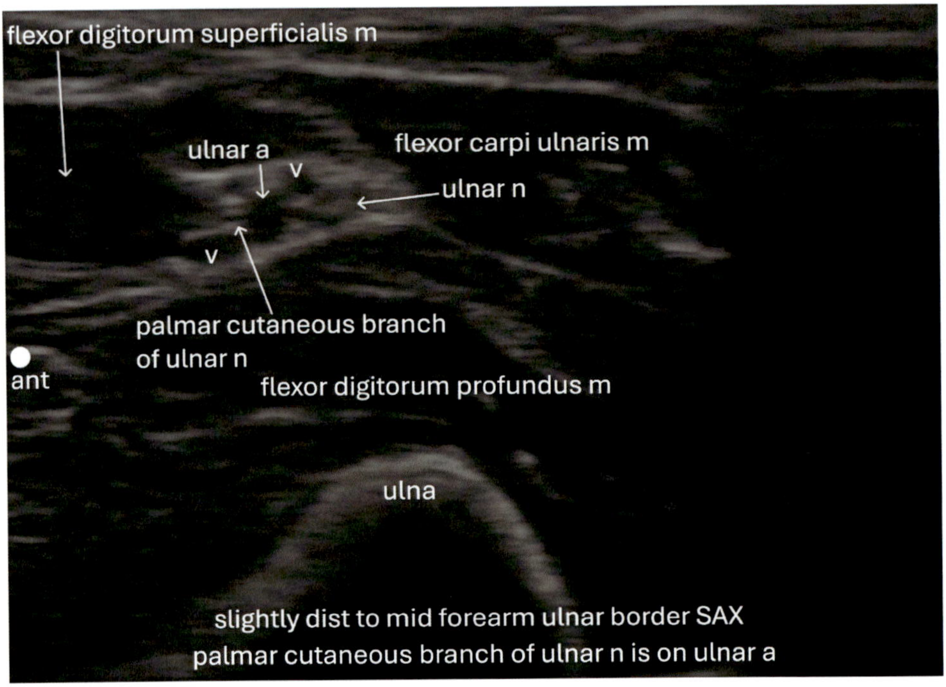

Probe Position: The probe is placed transversely on the ulnar border of the mid-forearm, just distal to the location shown in Fig. 11.

Anatomical Landmark: The ulnar artery.

Surrounding Structure: The ulnar nerve is situated just medial to the ulnar artery. The palmar cutaneous branch of the ulnar nerve may be visible on the lateral side of the ulnar artery. After this level, the palmar cutaneous branch of the ulnar nerve courses through the subcutaneous fat. It then passes superficial to the flexor retinaculum to provide sensation to the medial aspect of the palm.

Additional Observations: The flexor carpi ulnaris, the flexor digitorum superficialis, and the flexor digitorum profundus muscles are visible.

Fig. 13 Dorsal Cutaneous Branch of Ulnar Nerve / Ulnar Nerve / Flexor Carpi Ulnaris Muscle / Flexor Digitorum Superficialis and Profundus Muscles / Ulnar Artery / Pronator Quadratus Muscle

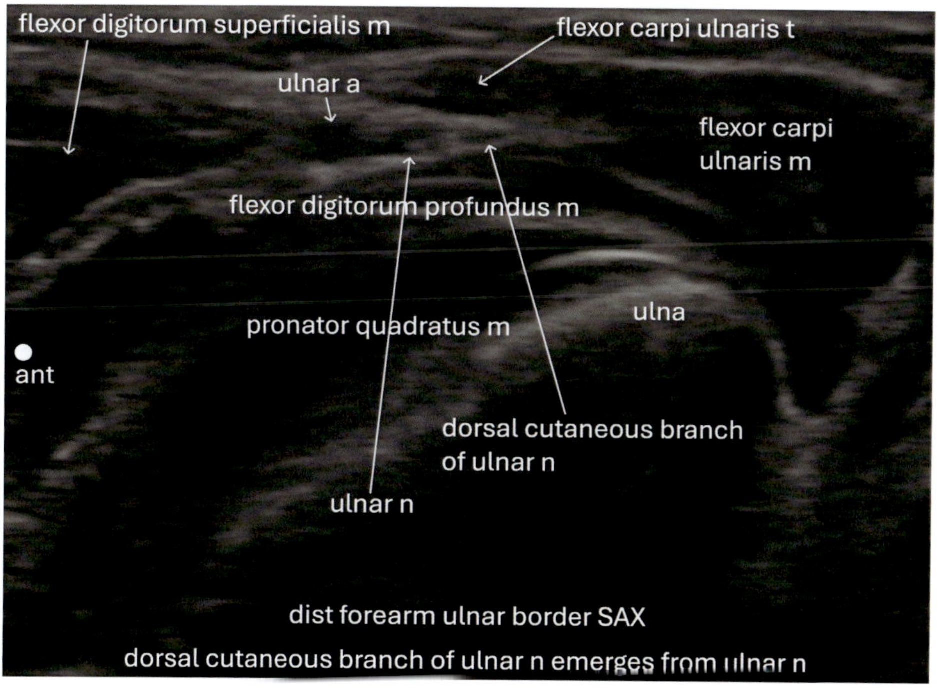

Probe Position: The probe is placed transversely on the ulnar border of the distal forearm, just distal to the location shown in Fig. 12.

Anatomical Landmarks: The ulnar artery, the flexor carpi ulnaris tendon, and the pronator quadratus muscle.

Surrounding Structures: The ulnar nerve is situated just medial to the ulnar artery. As the pronator quadratus muscle becomes visible deep to the flexor digitorum profundus muscle, the dorsal cutaneous branch of the ulnar nerve emerges from the ulnar nerve just deep to the tendon of the flexor carpi ulnaris muscle.

Additional Observation: The dorsal cutaneous branch of the ulnar nerve passes under the flexor carpi ulnaris muscle, heading medially as the probe is moved distally.

Fig. 14 Dorsal Cutaneous Branch of Ulnar Nerve / Ulnar Nerve / Flexor Carpi Ulnaris Muscle / Flexor Digitorum Superficialis and Profundus Muscles / Ulnar Artery / Pronator Quadratus Muscle

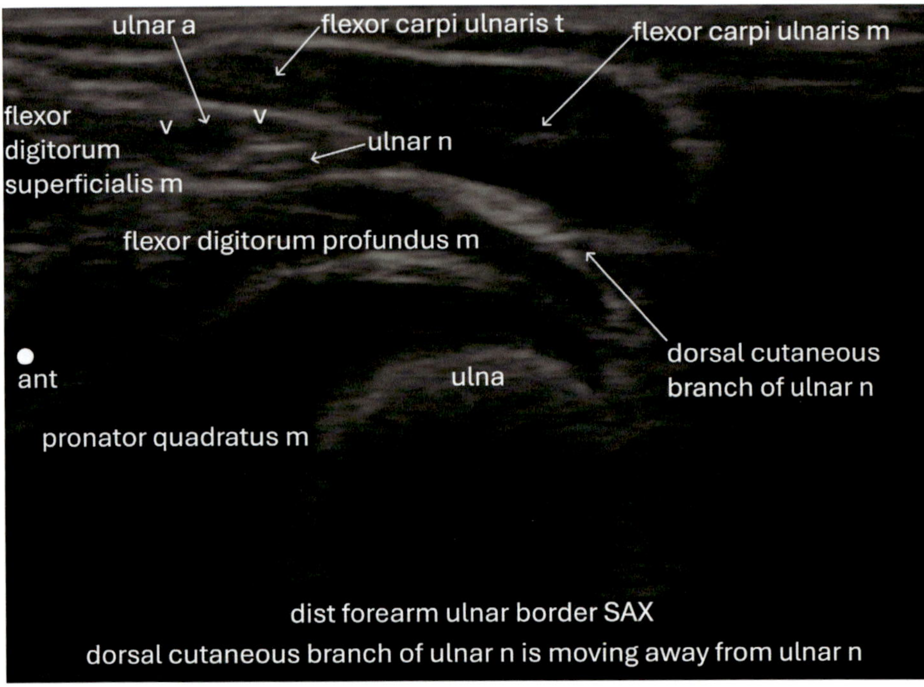

Probe Position: The probe is placed transversely on the ulnar border of the distal forearm, just distal to the location shown in Fig. 13.

Anatomical Landmarks: The ulnar artery, the flexor carpi ulnaris tendon, and the pronator quadratus muscle.

Surrounding Structures: The ulnar nerve is situated just medial to the ulnar artery under the flexor carpi ulnaris tendon. The dorsal cutaneous branch of the ulnar nerve travels deep to the flexor carpi ulnaris muscle, moving medially. As it courses distally, it spirals posteriorly around the ulna bone. It eventually pierces the deep antebrachial fascia to become subcutaneous.

Additional Observations: The flexor carpi ulnaris tendon and the pronator quadratus muscle are visible.

Fig. 15 Ulnar Nerve / Musculotendinous Junctions of Flexor Carpi Ulnaris, Flexor Digitorum Superficialis, and Flexor Digitorum Profundus / Ulnar Artery / Pronator Quadratus Muscle

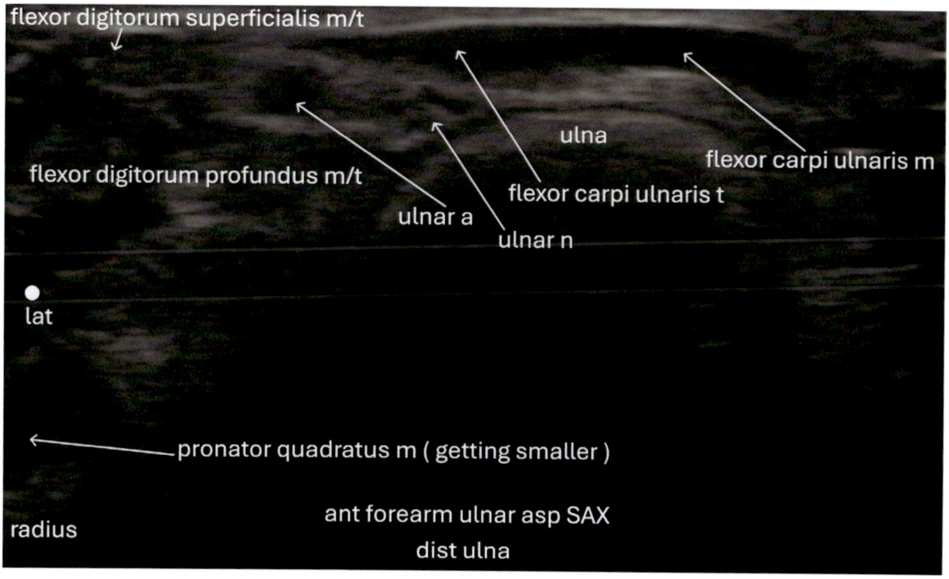

Probe Position: The probe is placed transversely on the ulnar side of the distal anterior forearm, just distal to the location shown in Fig. 14.

Anatomical Landmarks: The ulnar artery, the flexor carpi ulnaris tendon, and the pronator quadratus muscle.

Surrounding Structures: The ulnar nerve is situated medial to the ulnar artery and deep to the flexor carpi ulnaris tendon.

Additional Observations: The pronator quadratus muscle is visible on the radius, toward its insertion. The musculotendinous junctions of the flexor carpi ulnaris, the flexor digitorum superficialis, and the flexor digitorum profundus are visible.

Fig. 16 Ulnar Nerve / Musculotendinous Junctions of Flexor Carpi Ulnaris and Flexor Digitorum Superficialis / Flexor Digitorum Profundus Tendons / Ulnar Artery / Lunate / Triquetrum

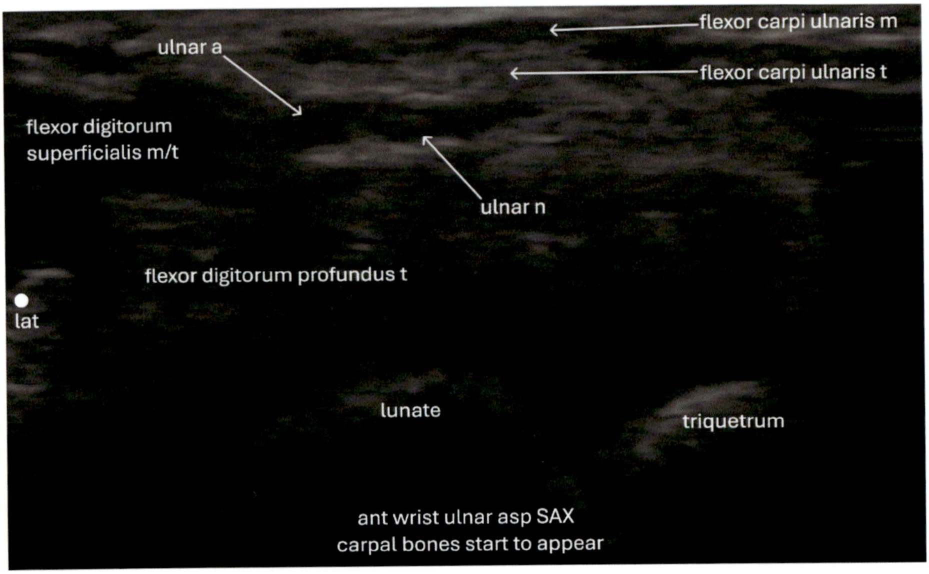

Probe Position: The probe is placed transversely on the ulnar side of the anterior wrist, just distal to the location shown in Fig. 15.

Anatomical Landmarks: The ulnar artery, the flexor carpi ulnaris tendon, the lunate, and the triquetrum.

Surrounding Structures: The ulnar nerve is located just medial to the ulnar artery and deep to the flexor carpi ulnaris tendon.

Additional Observations: The pronator quadratus muscle is no longer visible. The musculotendinous junctions of the flexor carpi ulnaris and the flexor digitorum superficialis are visible. The flexor digitorum profundus tendons are also visible. The carpal bones are beginning to appear.

Fig. 17 Ulnar Nerve / Tendons of Flexor Carpi Ulnaris, Flexor Digitorum Superficialis, and Flexor Digitorum Profundus / Ulnar Artery / Pisiform / Guyon's Canal

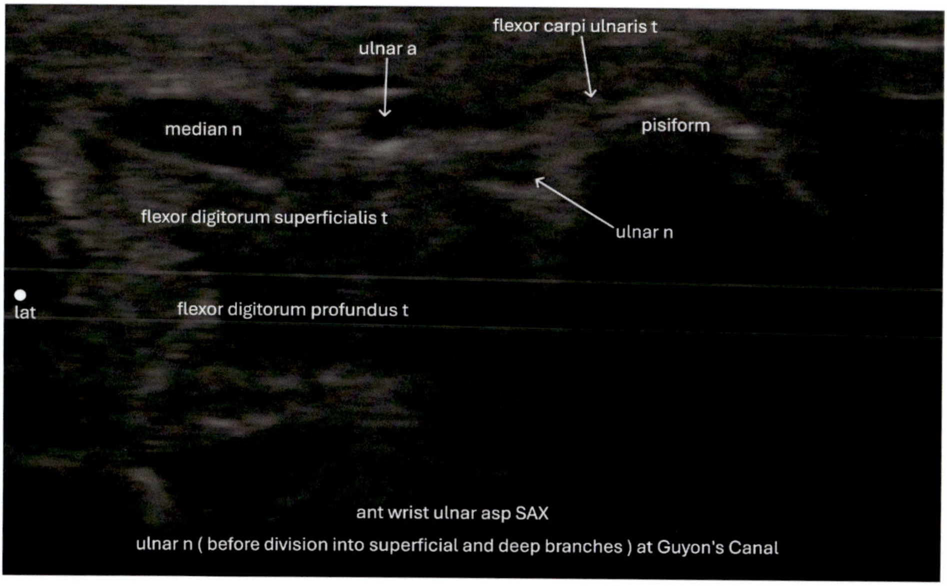

Probe Position: The probe is placed transversely on the ulnar side of the anterior wrist, just distal to the location shown in Fig. 16.

Anatomical Landmarks: The ulnar artery, the flexor carpi ulnaris tendon, and the pisiform.

Surrounding Structures: The ulnar nerve is located between the ulnar artery and the pisiform in Guyon's canal, beneath the insertion of the flexor carpi ulnaris tendon to the pisiform.

Additional Observations: The tendons of the flexor carpi ulnaris, the flexor digitorum superficialis, and the flexor digitorum profundus are visible. The median nerve is located lateral to the ulnar artery.

Fig. 18 Ulnar Nerve / Abductor Digiti Minimi Muscle / Ulnar Artery / Distal Pisiform / Guyon's Canal

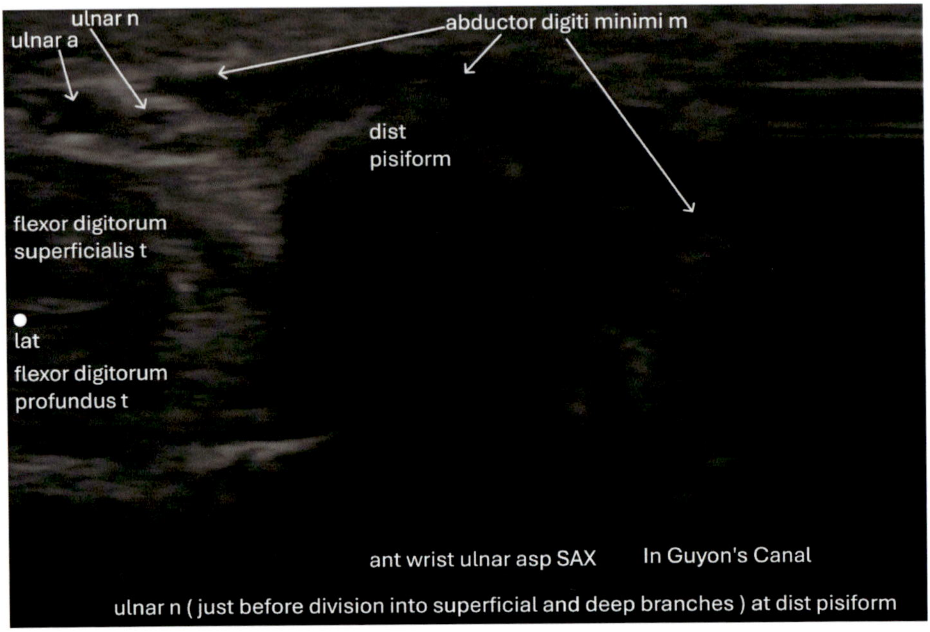

Probe Position: The probe is placed transversely on the ulnar side of the anterior wrist, just distal to the location shown in Fig. 17.

Anatomical Landmarks: The ulnar artery, the abductor digiti minimi muscle, and the distal portion of the pisiform bone.

Surrounding Structures: The ulnar nerve is located in Guyon's canal, between the ulnar artery and the distal portion of the pisiform bone. The abductor digiti minimi muscle is medial to the ulnar nerve and lies over the distal part of the pisiform bone. Its muscle belly extends further medially.

Additional Observation: The ulnar nerve will soon divide into a superficial and a deep branch.

Fig. 19 Superficial and Deep Branches of Ulnar Nerve / Abductor Digiti Minimi Muscle / Ulnar Artery / Level Just Distal to Pisiform Bone / Guyon's Canal

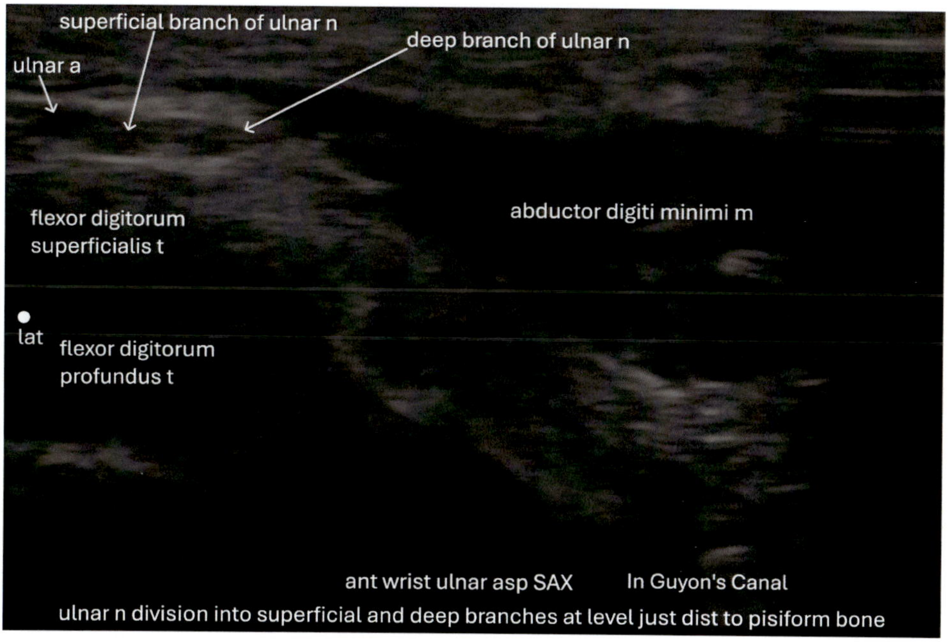

Probe Position: The probe is placed transversely on the ulnar side of the anterior wrist, just distal to the location shown in Fig. 18.

Anatomical Landmarks: The ulnar artery, the abductor digiti minimi muscle, and the region just distal to the pisiform bone.

Surrounding Structures: The ulnar nerve branches into a superficial and a deep branch. (Note that the level of this division can vary anatomically.) Both branches are located within Guyon's canal, situated between the ulnar artery and the abductor digiti minimi muscle.

Additional Observations: The flexor digitorum superficialis and profundus tendons are visible.

Fig. 20 Superficial and Deep Branches of Ulnar Nerve / Abductor Digiti Minimi Muscle / Ulnar Artery / Level Just Proximal to Hook of Hamate / Guyon's Canal

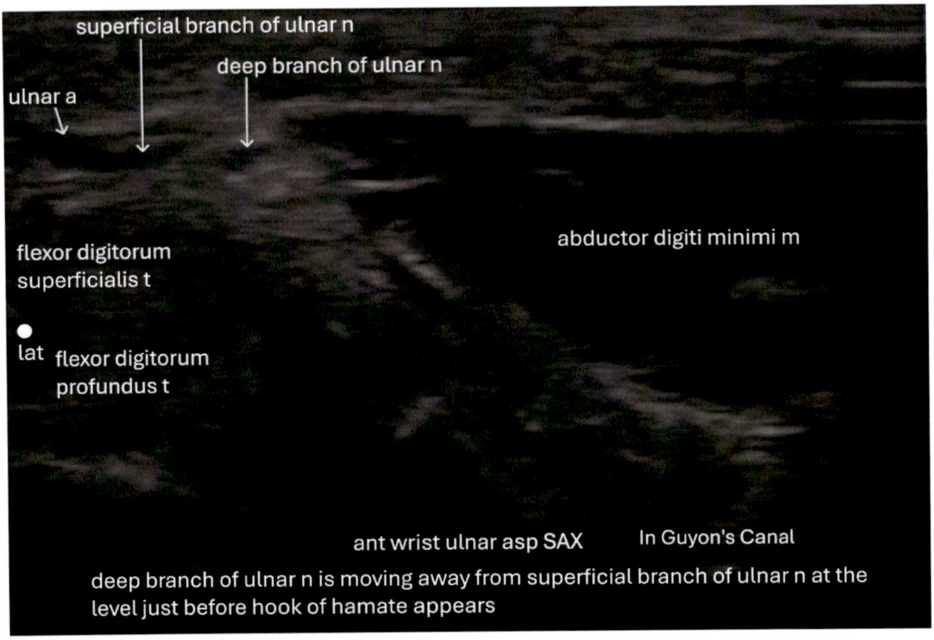

Probe Position: The probe is placed transversely on the ulnar side of the anterior wrist, just distal to the location shown in Fig. 19.

Anatomical Landmarks: The ulnar artery, the abductor digiti minimi muscle, and the region just proximal to the hook of hamate.

Surrounding Structures: Both the superficial and deep branches of the ulnar nerve are located within Guyon's canal, situated between the ulnar artery and the abductor digiti minimi muscle. The deep branch is positioned slightly away from the superficial branch.

Additional Observation: The hook of hamate will appear distally in a moment.

Fig. 21 Superficial and Deep Branches of Ulnar Nerve / Abductor Digiti Minimi Muscle / Ulnar Artery / Proximal Part of Hook of Hamate / Guyon's Canal / Flexor Digiti Minimi Brevis Muscle

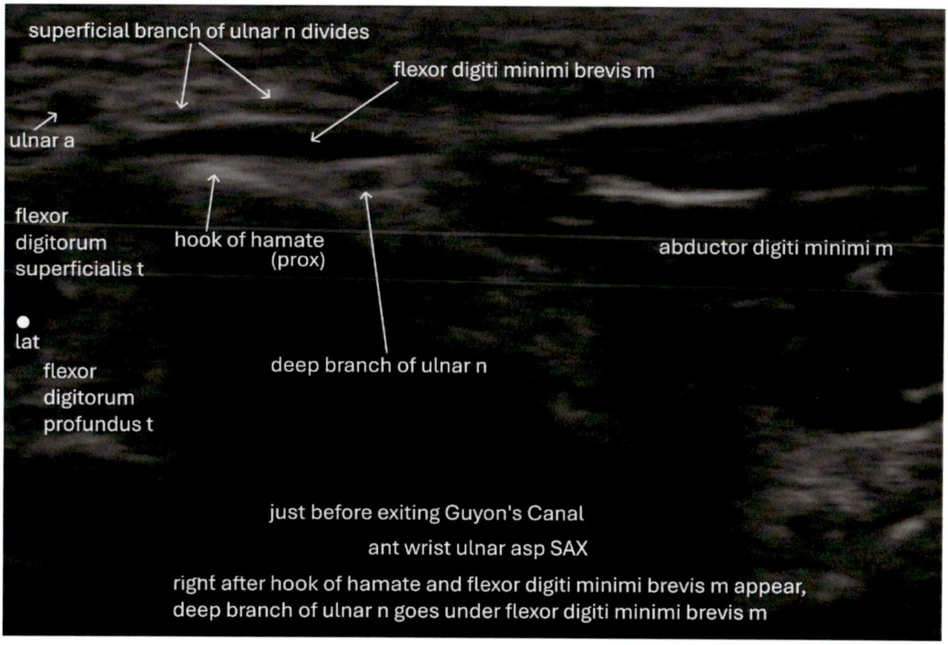

Probe Position: The probe is placed transversely on the ulnar side of the anterior wrist, just distal to the location shown in Fig. 20.

Anatomical Landmarks: The ulnar artery, the abductor digiti minimi muscle, the proximal part of the hook of hamate, and the flexor digiti minimi brevis muscle.

Surrounding Structures: Both the superficial and deep branches of the ulnar nerve are in the distal part of Guyon's canal, situated between the ulnar artery and the abductor digiti minimi muscle. The distal part of the canal is divided into a superficial and a deep compartment, each housing the corresponding nerve branch.

Additional Observations: In this view, the division of the superficial branch of the ulnar nerve is visible. The flexor digiti minimi brevis muscle begins to appear on the hook of hamate. The deep branch of the ulnar nerve courses deep to this muscle, while the superficial branch remains superficial.

Fig. 22 Deep Branch of Ulnar Nerve / Abductor Digiti Minimi Muscle / Distal Part of Hook of Hamate / Exit of Guyon's Canal / Flexor Digiti Minimi Brevis Muscle / Opponens Digiti Minimi Muscle

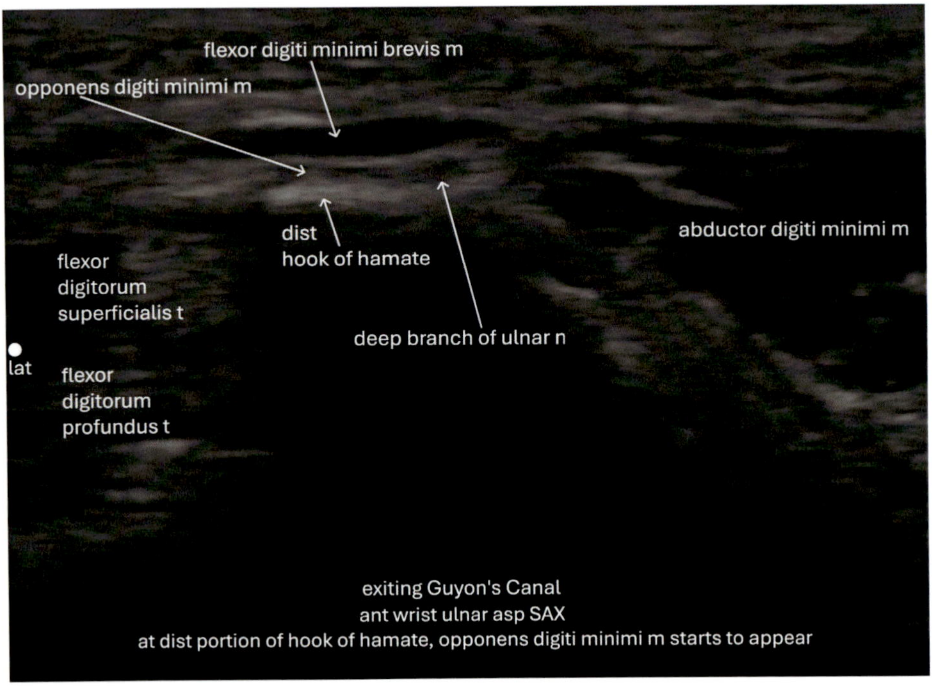

Probe Position: The probe is placed transversely on the ulnar side of the anterior wrist, just distal to the location shown in Fig. 21.

Anatomical Landmarks: The distal part of the hook of hamate and the flexor digiti minimi brevis muscle.

Surrounding Structure: At this level, both the superficial (not shown here) and deep branches of the ulnar nerve are at the exit of or exiting Guyon's canal.

Additional Observations: The opponens digiti minimi muscle begins to appear on the hook of hamate. The deep branch of the ulnar nerve is situated just medial to this muscle and deep to the flexor digiti minimi brevis muscle.

Fig. 23 Deep Branch of Ulnar Nerve / Abductor Digiti Minimi Muscle / Flexor Digiti Minimi Brevis Muscle / Opponens Digiti Minimi Muscle / 5th Metacarpal Base

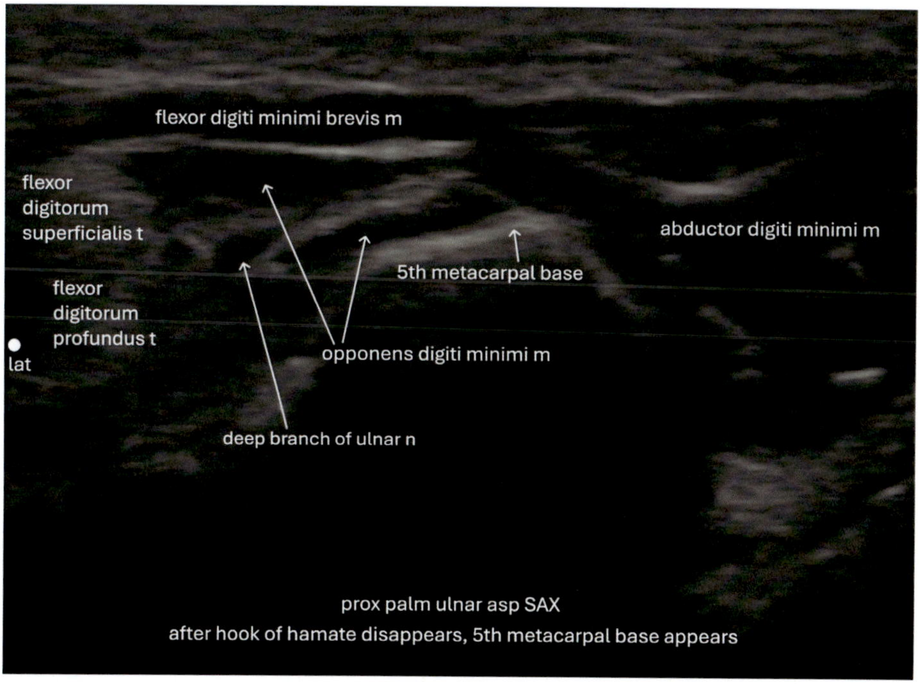

Probe Position: The probe is placed transversely on the ulnar side of the proximal palm, just distal to the location shown in Fig. 22.

Anatomical Landmarks: The fifth metacarpal base and the opponens digiti minimi muscle.

Surrounding Structures: At this level, the deep branch of the ulnar nerve runs along the deep surface of the opponens digiti minimi muscle, which lies over the fifth metacarpal. Then, it courses laterally across the deep palm, passing deep to the flexor tendons and coursing over the palmar surface of the interosseous muscles.

Additional Observation: Immediately after the hook of hamate disappears from view as the probe is moved inferiorly, the fifth metacarpal bone begins to appear slightly medial to the hook of hamate.

Fig. 24 Abductor Digiti Minimi Muscle / Flexor Digiti Minimi Brevis Muscle / Opponens Digiti Minimi Muscle / Proximal 5th Metacarpal / Palmar Interosseous Muscle

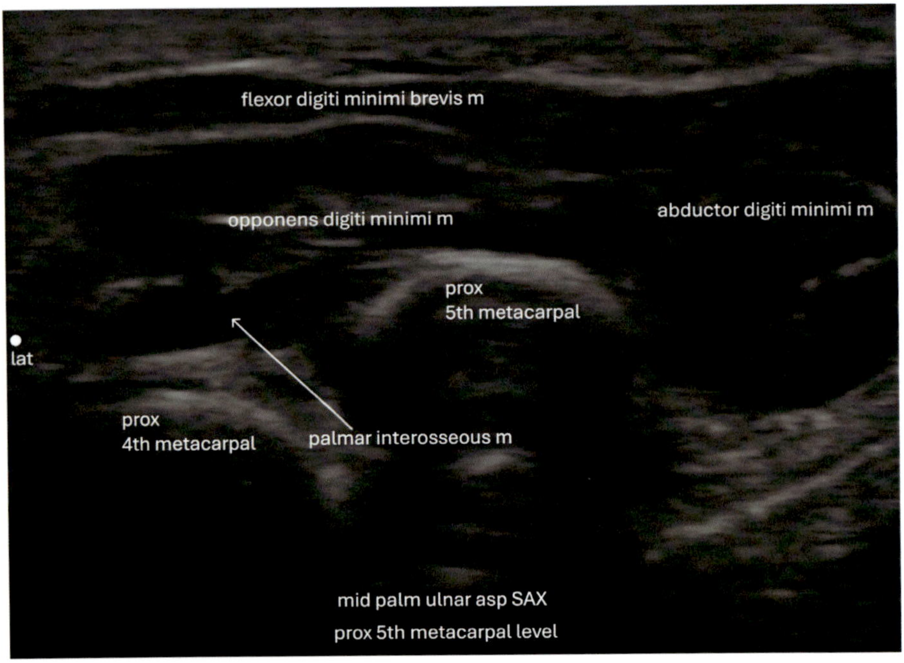

Probe Position: The probe is placed transversely on the ulnar side of the mid-palm, just distal to the position shown in Fig. 23.

Anatomical Landmarks: The fourth and fifth metacarpals.

Visualized Structures: The palmar interosseous muscle appears on the radial side of the proximal portion of the fifth metacarpal.

Additional Observations: The abductor digiti minimi, flexor digiti minimi brevis, and opponens digiti minimi muscles are visible.

Fig. 25 Abductor Digiti Minimi Muscle / Flexor Digiti Minimi Brevis Muscle / Opponens Digiti Minimi Muscle / Mid-5th Metacarpal / Palmar and Dorsal Interosseous Muscles

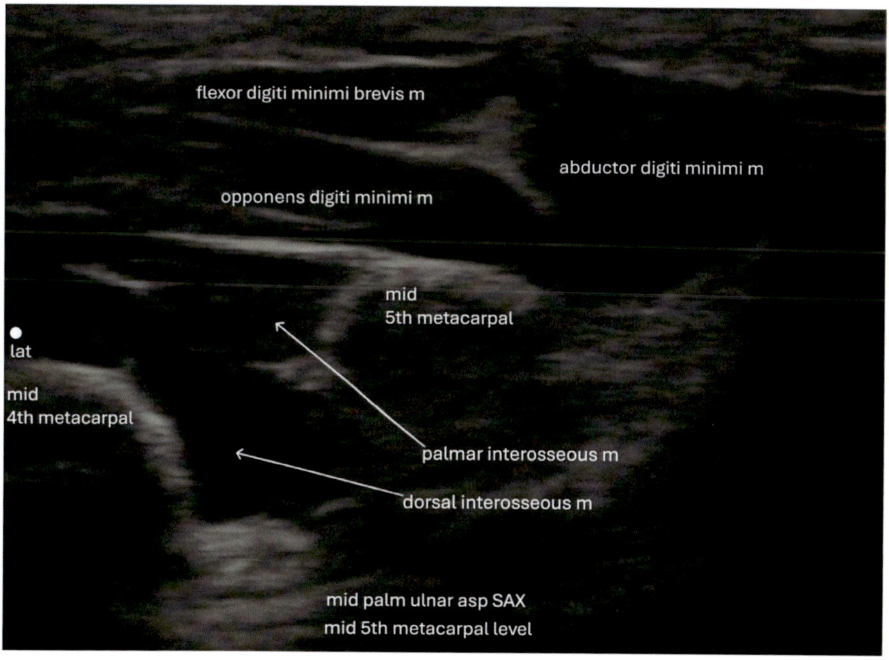

Probe Position: The probe is placed transversely on the ulnar side of the mid-palm, just distal to the position shown in Fig. 24.

Anatomical Landmarks: The fourth and fifth metacarpals.

Visualized Structures: The dorsal interosseous muscle is visible between the mid-portion of the fourth and fifth metacarpals, deep (posterior) to the palmar interosseous muscle.

Additional Observations: The abductor digiti minimi, flexor digiti minimi brevis, and opponens digiti minimi muscles are visible.

Fig. 26 Abductor Digiti Minimi Muscle / Flexor Digiti Minimi Brevis Muscle / Opponens Digiti Minimi Muscle / Neck of 5th Metacarpal / Palmar and Dorsal Interosseous Muscles

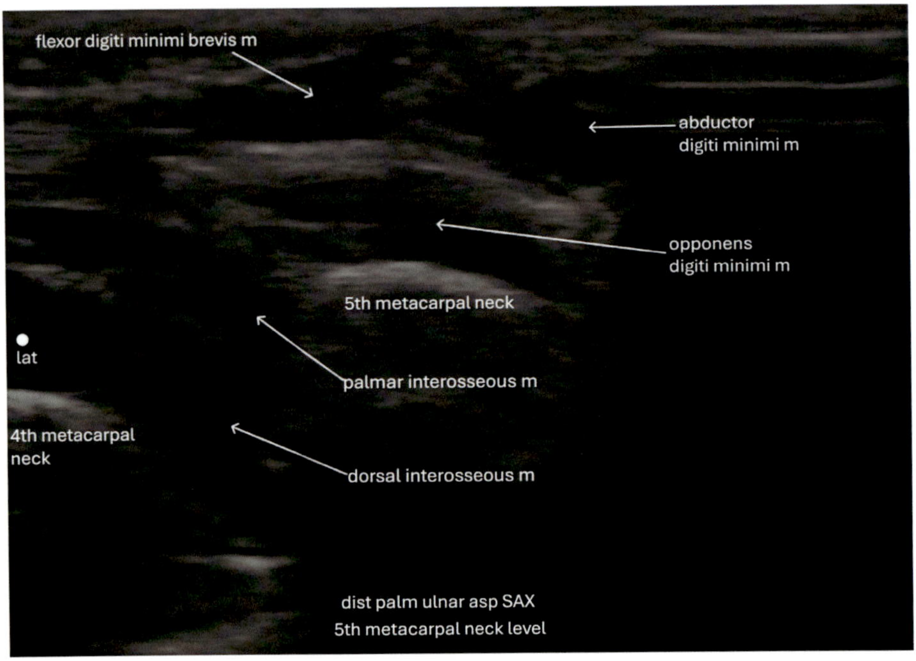

Probe Position: The probe is placed transversely on the ulnar side of the distal palm, just distal to the position shown in Fig. 25.

Anatomical Landmarks: The fourth and fifth metacarpals.

Visualized Structures: The dorsal interosseous muscle is visible between the neck of the fourth and fifth metacarpals, deep (posterior) to the palmar interosseous muscle.

Additional Observation: The abductor digiti minimi, flexor digiti minimi brevis, and opponens digiti minimi muscles are visible superficial to the neck of the fifth metacarpal, tapering distally.

Fig. 27 Abductor Digiti Minimi Muscle / Flexor Digiti Minimi Brevis Muscle / Head of 5th Metacarpal

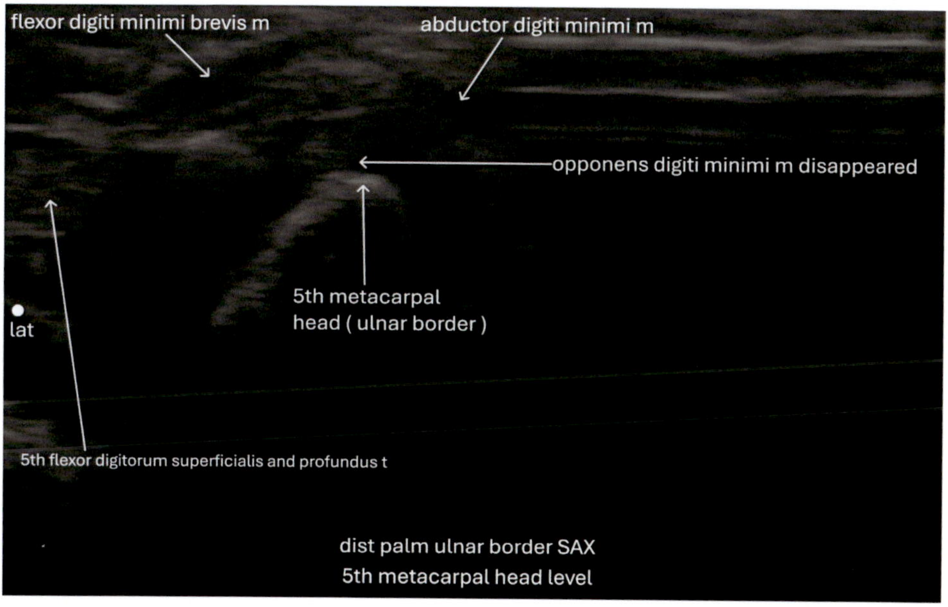

Probe Position: The probe is placed transversely on the ulnar border of the distal palm, just distal to the position shown in Fig. 26.

Anatomical Landmark: The ulnar border of the head of the fifth metacarpal.

Visualized Structures: The opponens digiti minimi inserts along the ulnar side of the shaft of the fifth metacarpal, extending distally toward the head, and is no longer visible in this view. The abductor digiti minimi and flexor digiti minimi brevis taper as they approach their insertions.

Additional Observation: The flexor digitorum superficialis and profundus tendons for the fifth digit can be seen in the left portion of the image.

Fig. 28 Anterior Ulnar Aspect of Base of Proximal Phalanx of 5th Digit

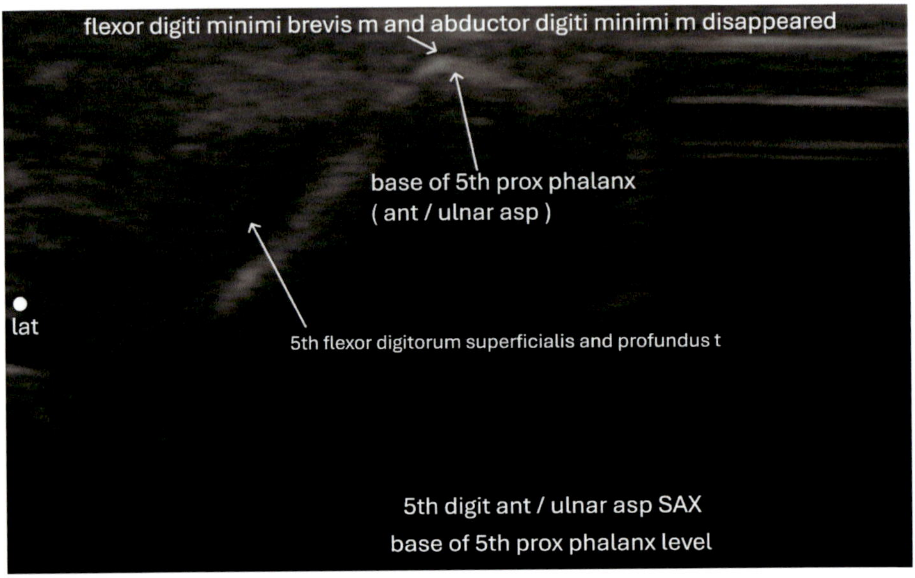

Probe Position: The probe is placed transversely on the anterior ulnar aspect of the proximal fifth finger, just distal to the position shown in Fig. 27.

Anatomical Landmark: The anterior ulnar aspect of the base of the proximal phalanx of the fifth digit.

Visualized Structure: As the abductor digiti minimi and flexor digiti minimi brevis taper toward their insertions, they are no longer visible in this view. Their insertion is located on the anterior ulnar aspect of the base of the proximal phalanx of the fifth digit. They share this common bony insertion, although the abductor digiti minimi may also contribute fibers to the extensor expansion.

Additional Observation: The flexor digitorum superficialis and profundus tendons for the fifth digit can be seen lateral to this insertion site.

www.ingramcontent.com/pod-product-compliance
Ingram Content Group UK Ltd.
Pitfield, Milton Keynes, MK11 3LW, UK
UKRC040218051026
15591UKWH00011B/361

9781764437707

9 781764 437707